YOUNGER SKIN

YOUNGER SKIN

How to Get It, How to Keep It

Jonathan Zizmor, M.D.,
and Sharon Sabin

HOLT, RINEHART AND WINSTON // NEW YORK

First published in January 1984 by Holt, Rinehart and Winston,
383 Madison Avenue, New York, New York 10017.
Published simultaneously in Canada by Holt, Rinehart and Winston
of Canada, Limited.

Library of Congress Cataloging in Publication Data
Zizmor, Jonathan.
Younger skin.
Includes index.
1. Skin—Care and hygiene.   2. Skin—Diseases—
Treatment.   3. Skin—Aging.   I. Sabin, Sharon. II. Ti-
tle.
RC87.Z48   1983   646.7′26   83-4398
ISBN: 0-03-061577-1

FIRST EDITION

Designer: *Debra L. Moloshok*
Printed in the United States of America
1 2 3 4 5 6 7 8 9 10

ISBN 0-03-061577-1

CONTENTS

YOUNGER SKIN

INTRODUCTION

Looking young has become a national obsession in our youth-oriented, affluent society. Everyone is preoccupied with maintaining or restoring a perennially youthful appearance.

Prominent personalities boast about their face-lifts on television talk shows, while housewives stalk the aisles of Bloomingdale's in hot pursuit of the latest miracle cream for their skin. There is ample evidence that men and women in America today are spending a good deal of time and hundreds of millions of dollars a year in a frantic effort to delay or reverse the onslaught of aging.

The motivation behind all this activity is clear. No one wants to grow old in a culture that equates youth with desirability. Men and women alike strive to be socially attractive and economically marketable for as long as possible.

For many years, well-heeled magnates, jet-set-

1

ting socialites, and famous entertainers have been seeking medical help to erase the telltale signs of aging. Others with financial means and the same goals would gladly do likewise if only they knew what could be done and how to go about doing it. The concern with arresting the ravages of time is virtually universal.

Recent medical advances have made it feasible to grow old and still look young. In fact, the once impossible dream is both available and affordable now that there are medically proven, safe ways to achieve, restore, and maintain a youthful appearance.

What is not readily at hand, however, is information that spells out exactly what can be done, how much treatments cost, and where you can find the medical help to do them. That's where this book comes in. Designed to fill the information gap, this book provides a definitive, practical guide to the new types of rejuvenating medical treatments and revolutionary products that are available to help you regain and preserve younger-looking skin without undergoing plastic surgery.

In these pages, you will find out what you can do for deep lines and wrinkles that make you look and feel old. There are chapters on each of the three highly effective injection therapies—collagen, silicone, and fibrin foam—that describe in detail what you can expect to experience, the risks that are involved, the chances of success, and how the therapies work. The pros and cons of the three treatments are examined in terms of cost, efficacy, short-term and long-term health hazards, and the relative importance of the skill of the attending physician.

Here, too, you will discover what can be done for blotchy, rough, or unevenly textured sun-damaged skin that gives away your age or makes you appear older than you are. There are chapters on revolutionary topical medications—Retin-A and Efudex—that literally resurface skin and restore its youthful appearance. These chapters explain how the preparations work and include practical tips on ways you can apply them prophylactically and care for your skin to keep it from aging.

You will learn about the medical remedies that can correct bothersome tiny lines, fine crevices, or other minor facial imperfections that spoil your otherwise youthful appearance. There are chapters on electronic facials and other nonsurgical skin treatments, chemical abrasions and dermabrasions, as well as a chapter devoted to over-the-counter products you can buy to protect your skin from damaging solar rays, keep it moist and soft, and cover up its defects. Finally, there are specific, step-by-step regimens to follow to restore your skin to its maximum youthful potential.

By reading the chapters that follow, you will not only familiarize yourself with all that is now medically possible to make you look younger but also glean everything you need to know to take advantage of the latest medical advances, including how to go about getting the best doctor for your treatment of choice. You'll come away armed with all the knowledge you need to confidently select the help you want at a price you can afford to treat yourself to younger skin.

1   INJECTING A FACE-LIFT

Do not be self-conscious about those telltale lines and wrinkles that are beginning to appear on your face. If such signs of advancing age are getting you down or making you unhappy, depressed, or dissatisfied with yourself, you *can* do something about them without undertaking painful disrupting surgery or incurring huge expense. The answer: two or several injections of a revolutionary new substance— Zyderm. It is safe, painless, and highly effective. The result: a virtual face-lift after a couple or more injections, without having to undergo an operation.

Reasonably priced and affordable, Zyderm is widely available through doctors almost everywhere in the United States. Certified and approved by the Food and Drug Administration (FDA) in 1981 as a safe medical device after exhaustive research and testing, this miracle boon to youth preservation can achieve remarkable improvements. Embarrassing facial furrows and crags, unsightly depressions—and even some acne scars—can be filled in and erased, making skin appear smoother and younger-looking. The noticeable physical change could make a critical psychological difference.

What Zyderm Is and How It Works

Zyderm is a highly purified form of collagen, a natural protein that provides the structural support and framework for skin and other soft tissues in humans and animals. Collagen is the scaffolding that props skin up and fills it out, keeping it taut and firm. When facial collagen disintegrates, withers, or collapses with age, skin sags, sinks, and falls into lines, wrinkles, and other depressions. How soon or fast this happens depends on an individual's heredity and facial habits. A person who continuously animates his features a certain way—smiles or frowns a lot—may find to his dismay that such expressiveness eventually leaves indelible impressions on his face as he gets older.

Studies have revealed that there is very little difference in the composition of collagen—either among various persons or between human beings and other animals. That is why Zyderm—which is prepared from cattle skin that has been specially processed to remove all suspect or extraneous materials—closely mimics human collagen.

Because of its similarity to human collagen and the fact that collagen occurs naturally in human skin, Zyderm is the perfect injectable substance, usually readily absorbed without any side effects. It is interesting to note, too, that although the Zyderm implant itself is relatively new, other animal collagen products—such as artificial heart valves and stitching sutures—that have been inserted in humans and utilized as medical devices have a long track record of performing safely and effectively for many years.

Zyderm is injected *into* the skin, not under it. A natural substance that is natural to the skin itself, the Zyderm-collagen is rapidly incorporated into the facial support tissue and becomes an integral part of it, propping up the sags and crags—the wrinkles and lines—where the facial skin's own collagen has given way or disintegrated. Within weeks, the surrounding tissue wraps itself around the newfound framework, encapsulating the Zyderm-collagen implant so completely that it cannot be distinguished from the body's own natural collagen.

The Zyderm-collagen implant is injected with a very fine, 30-gauge needle, which doesn't leave a noticeable mark. The simple procedure—each injection no more complicated than a flu shot—can be done in a doctor's office over a lunch hour. Depending on the particular condition to be corrected, between two and six injections usually suffice to achieve the desired level of improvement. Treatment sessions generally last no more than a half hour and are spaced at least two weeks apart.

An injectable soft-tissue replacement for the body's deficient collagen supports, Zyderm fills in depressed areas and raises the skin to the level of the surrounding tissue. Zyderm implants can correct a wide range of soft-tissue defects—frown and smile furrows, crevices, wrinkles, lines, sunken areas, and minor scars—and at the same time soften scar tissue and improve skin texture. A viable alternative to surgery that involves only a brief in-office procedure with minimal recovery time, Zyderm-collagen implants are a safe, effective, and convenient way to make someone look better and/or younger.

What Zyderm Can Do for You

Zyderm treatments do not entail a lot of time, fuss, bother, or discomfort. Nor do they involve a great expense. Total costs for correcting minimal wrinkles or scars run between $500 and $700, depending on the nature and extent of the condition treated, while fees for improving deep maximal or widespread scars and wrinkles range between $2000 and $3000.

In considering Zyderm treatments, it is vitally important to stress the need for realistic assessments about what is possible in the way of improvement. As with all cosmetic therapy, the cardinal rule is: Don't expect to look very different, just somewhat better.

Zyderm-collagen implants work best for certain types of defects. Grosser lines are more easily corrected than finer ones. The same goes for wrinkles. The more noticeable the defect, the more effective and satisfying to the patient the treatment is likely to be.

Deep frown and smile furrows running vertically down the cheeks respond well to Zyderm therapy, as do sunken areas resulting from natural atrophy, disease, injury, or surgical mishaps. Very fine horizontal lines on the forehead and tiny aging lines around the mouth are difficult to correct.

Creases and folds on the neck caused by excess skin are not at all suited to Zyderm therapy. Zyderm implant use is prohibited for breast augmentation.

As far as scars are concerned, those that are soft and movable are more likely to be improved by Zyderm-collagen implants than those that are hard or have very sharp margins, such as pockmarks, or "ice pick" acne scars, which are very difficult to correct. However, even with these latter scar types, some success has been reported using Zyderm if the first implant is injected directly into the scar itself to soften it and then subsequent Zyderm implants are put into place within the softened area.

For the various soft-tissue defects described above—gross lines and wrinkles, deep smile or frown furrows, sunken areas, and certain scars—Zyderm-collagen renders significant improvements by raising depressed facial tissue to surrounding contour levels and evening out skin texture. The resulting overall impression is that the face appears smoother, tauter, more attractive, and younger-looking.

The only aftereffect of a Zyderm-collagen implant is a slight swelling, which disappears within a day or two. As a matter of fact, if some swelling is not present it is likely that you won't see any improvement. The reason for this is that the key to successful Zyderm therapy is *overcorrection*. Because the injected fluid's volume is composed largely of water and lidocaine—an anesthetic similar to novocaine—and contains relatively little collagen, the inflammation disappears rapidly as the liquid is absorbed into the body. Only the small amount of collagen leaves a lasting impression. So, if the treated area doesn't appear bumpy and/or swollen for some time after the injection, that is more cause for concern than not. It means one of two things. Either you received no collagen at all in the injection, or you received not enough to make it worthwhile.

This can happen because not all doctors have access to Zyderm implants. The ones that do are selected and supplied by Zyderm's manufacturer—Collagen Corporation of Palo Alto, California—which strictly regulates and monitors its use.

To make sure you get the real McCoy when you

go for Zyderm-collagen injections, insist that your doctor open the syringe in front of you. Each one bears the Zyderm trademark as well as a specific identification number and date and is labeled according to dosage contents. That way you will know if, and how much, genuine Zyderm is being shot into you. Also, keep in mind that for Zyderm to be fully effective, it requires refrigeration. If you see that the injection syringe has not been kept in cold storage, demand a replacement, an explanation, or both.

Getting Zyderm Therapy

If you want to consult a dermatologist or plastic surgeon about the possibility of getting Zyderm implant treatments, your best bet is to write to the Collagen Corporation to obtain the names of physicians in your area who are supplied with the material. Doctors who receive Zyderm syringes are registered with the company and must follow a set procedure. Here is what you can expect if you consult one of these physicians about a Zyderm implant.

First you will be provided with a patient-information booklet that explains the benefits and potential complications and risks involved in undertaking this type of treatment. If, after reading this booklet through, you decide you want to go ahead, you will be asked to complete a detailed questionnaire on your medical history, which is designed to screen out those patients who are likely to react negatively to Zyderm-collagen therapy.

Certain prior medical conditions *per se* rule out the possibility of having Zyderm injections. If you have ever had a personal or family history of lupus, rheumatoid arthritis or related diseases, allergic reactions, or if you have a sensitivity to lidocaine or novocaine, you are ineligible to proceed with Zyderm. A record of any autoimmune disease—such as ulcerative colitis, polymyositis, Reiter's Syndrome, or sclerosis—among your immediate relatives also disqualifies you from receiving Zyderm-collagen implants.

If, on the basis of the questionnaire and the type of facial defects you have, you qualify as a good candidate for Zyderm-collagen therapy, the doctor must administer a preliminary sensitivity test to make sure you are not allergic to the Zyderm-collagen mixture itself before the actual treatment can begin. (Remember to look for the Zyderm trademark on the test syringe.) After a small amount of the substance is injected into your forearm, you will be asked to wait four weeks to see if you have an adverse response. If no skin reaction—swelling, redness, soreness, or sensitivity—appears at the test site during that time, you will then be able to initiate your Zyderm treatment.

As indicated earlier, depending on the condition

to be corrected, you will receive between two and six Zyderm-collagen injections to achieve the desired level of improvement. After each treatment session, you can expect to experience a slight localized swelling—similar to that produced by a mosquito bite—accompanied by mild soreness and redness at the implant site. This is normal and should subside within twenty-four hours. Any swelling around your lips, however, may take somewhat longer to disappear.

On occasion, during the course of treatment, temporary bruising or discoloration may appear on the implant site. These reactions, too, are short-lived, and vanish after a few hours or a couple of days at most.

Besides the immediate reduction in swelling, some further loss of the contour correction achieved by the Zyderm-collagen injection can be expected over the first few weeks following the implant. But subsequent treatment sessions can compensate for this by putting into place additional layers of Zyderm-collagen until the final contour level proves satisfactory.

Interestingly enough, any dissatisfaction from Zyderm-collagen treatments usually is the result of a doctor "low-balling" the patient. This happens when the physician doesn't give the patient enough Zyderm-collagen in each individual injection he administers, or when he underestimates the number of injections required to achieve the desired level of improvement. In either case, such physicians are not overcorrecting sufficiently to make Zyderm therapy worthwhile.

As stated earlier, overcorrecting is vitally important to the success of Zyderm-collagen therapy. Only 25 to 30 percent of the fluid volume implanted by the Zyderm-collagen injection remains at the site as collagen support material to prop up sagging tissue. So substantial overcorrection is called for to achieve optimal results.

In practical terms, this means that if a doctor injects a quantity of Zyderm-collagen sufficient to produce an immediate correction to 60 percent of the normal contour, the patient ultimately will be left with a correction amounting to 15 percent of the normal contour. However, if the doctor injects enough Zyderm-collagen to yield an overcorrection of 150 percent, the patient will see eventual correction approaching 50 percent. Two or three such injections should result in total or 100 percent correction and restore the normal facial contour.

According to available reports, the overwhelming majority of patients who have received Zyderm implants have been extremely satisfied with the results. The safety record to date—with clinical data on more than 5000 persons who have undergone Zyderm therapy—indicates an adverse reaction rate of less than 2 percent.

Most adverse reactions—occasional firmness

at the implant site and swelling of the surrounding tissue—last only a few hours and usually are associated with consumption of alcohol, prolonged exposure to the sun and/or heat, and flare-ups of hay fever and other causes of nasal and sinus congestion. Reports indicate that these reactions haven't affected the long-term success of Zyderm-collagen implant corrections. Nevertheless, if you are having a series of Zyderm injections, you should avoid excessive exposure to the sun and minimize your intake of alcoholic beverages during the course of the treatments. Both sunbathing and social drinking may be enjoyed in moderation.

In rare cases—one out of a thousand—a patient has become sensitized to the Zyderm-collagen implant as a result of treatment. This type of allergic response, which produces redness and swelling at the implant sites, disappears within a couple of weeks. Also, be aware that if you previously have had a herpes infection on the implant site, there is a chance that the Zyderm-collagen injection could precipitate another herpes eruption.

Needless to say, the implantation of Zyderm-collagen carries an inherent—albeit minimal—risk of infection, as does any injection procedure. Before a treatment, be sure to wash your face thoroughly with soap and water. If you wear makeup, you can reapply it to the implant site a few hours after the injection. Use of Zyderm-collagen on facial areas where there is

15

an active skin eruption—such as a cyst, pimple, rash, or hive—should be postponed until the trouble has cleared.

Long-term Efficacy and Consequences

Since Zyderm-collagen is a newly developed substance that has been in use in cosmetic therapy for less than ten years, there is no hard clinical data on its long-term efficacy. Whether the corrections produced on the faces of the patients who have received the treatment will be permanent—or how long they will last if they are not—is still undetermined.

According to available reports, at least half of all Zyderm-collagen patients require no further injections up to three years after their treatment has ceased. However, the Collagen Corporation advises participating physicians to counsel all patients to expect some supplemental injections in order to maintain the optimal level of correction. After all, it is unrealistic to presume that the aging process will not take its toll on the Zyderm-collagen implant once it has become an integral part of the human body. Consequently, you should expect the change in correction over time to be about the same as the changes observed in the natural tissue at the implant site. And, if the condition that caused the soft-tissue depression—excessive frowning, for example—persists, it is likely that the defect will reappear sooner. To see whether you need maintenance therapy—a touch-up injection to implant somewhere between 10 and 20 percent more collagen—you should get yourself checked every six months or so.

As of this writing, a more potent version of Zyderm called Zyderm II has just been approved by the FDA. The advantage of using Zyderm II is that more significant improvements can be achieved without having to overcorrect as much. Consequently, the course of treatment is shorter and a lesser quantity of the injectable substance is required. The results are both quicker and better.

Because Zyderm-collagen therapy has been in use for such a short period of time, there is no significant data on its long-term consequences. However, while there is nothing in the clinical evidence to date to indicate that Zyderm-collagen implants are potentially hazardous in any way, it is a relatively new drug and should be used with caution by patient and physician.

2   FILLING IN

For deep wrinkles and age-revealing lines that mar your face and make you look older than you would like, there is an alternative to the relatively new and still somewhat experimental Zyderm-collagen treatment. It is a substance that has been in use for more than twenty years by qualified physicians on thousands of satisfied patients without any ill effects or troublesome consequences.

Like Zyderm-collagen, the treatment involves only a few uncomplicated injections that are virtually painless, trouble-free, and inexpensive. Highly effective for eliminating unsightly facial defects—smile creases, frown crags, and contour sags—this substance not only works remarkably well but also has a dependable track record of proven safety and long-lasting results.

Despite its unjustified bad reputation, the substance we are talking about—silicone—is an excellent therapeutic performer in the right hands. Any reported health-harming problems involving silicone in the past resulted from its misuse or adulteration by therapists who weren't properly qualified or skilled enough to administer it.

Background and Development of Silicone

For about a century, surgeons around the world have been looking for suitable materials to replace human body tissues lost or destroyed through atrophy, disease, accident, or mishap. During this time, a wide range of natural substances derived from animal, vegetable, and mineral sources has been tested as implants in human bodies. None of them proved ideal for the purpose, however.

Ivory and various metals (inserted in some patients in the early 1900s to reconstruct missing or deficient bone and cartilage tissue) and paraffin and lanolin (lodged in other patients to compensate for sagging tissue) all have been shown to produce negative reactions within the human body. Immediate or eventual complications—such as infections, allergic responses, serious illnesses, systemic traumas, granuloma formations (a severe skin reaction), cancers, blood disorders, and other dire consequences—appeared in an alarming number of cases involving these implanted substances. Because of this, such materials no longer are employed as medical implants here in the United States.

Still, the search for perfect implantable tissue substitutes continues. What doctors are after are substances with an unusual combination of properties. In fact, to be an acceptable and viable human-tissue implant, a substance needs to meet all or most of the following prerequisites.

Inertness is an especially important attribute. An implant material that is both chemically and physically inert is less likely to precipitate any disruptive changes within the human body.

In order to insure against ultimate rejection or expulsion, the implant substance must have a built-in compatibility with human tissue. That means it should be free of any toxic properties that could upset or disrupt the vital systems within the human body. Needless to say, it should not be a cancer-causing agent, or carcinogen.

As a safeguard against immediate or subsequent reactions, the substance itself must be impervious to change within the human body environment. To maintain its stability, the substance must be unaffected by time, heat, or pressure. Another vital requirement is that it should not support bacterial growth that could lead to infection. It also should be locally nonreactive to minimize temporary discomfort and flare-ups at the implant site.

Practically speaking, it is preferable for an im-

plant material to be both easy to sterilize and to prepare. And it is also desirable that it be inexpensive, if
possible, to promote widespread accessibility and
medical usage wherever and whenever needed.

Surprisingly enough, the most effective and in-
nocuous substances for medical implantation in humans that have been discovered so far are synthetic
creations, many of which were intended originally for
other purposes. Certain man-made plastics—such as
Teflon, Dacron, and some acrylics—that have been
enlisted and adapted as medical implants have proven
themselves to be top-performing, trouble-free bone
substitutes. At the same time, two processed injectable fluids—Zyderm-collagen and silicone, developed
here and abroad—are gaining widespread accept-
ance among the medical community as safe, effective
soft-tissue replacements well-suited to human implantation.

Silicone was the pathbreaker, capturing world-
wide attention when it was first introduced during
the late 1940s and early 1950s by European doctors
in headline-producing breast-ballooning operations
on notable and would-be famous actresses. Unfortunately, as was revealed later, the debut was in-
auspicious, since such procedures proved to be a
misapplication of this form of silicone.

Liquid silicone never was intended to be injected
directly into the breasts, especially in large quantities.
Principally suited to correcting facial defects, injec-

tions of silicone fluid work best when administered in very small amounts that are carefully meted out in a prescribed series.

Use of silicone to build up breasts is perfectly safe—if the silicone fluid is sealed within specially prepared rubberlike sacks, called *silastics*. This form of silicone can be safely implanted surgically in the chest cavity.

The silastic containers prevent problematic leakage and migration of the silicone liquid, the chief causes of the traumatic upsets, granulomas, and cancers experienced by many of the patients who had large doses of silicone fluid injected into their breasts to enlarge them.

Silicone fluid, when injected properly, does not migrate. Past problems can be attributed either to administering too much silicone liquid at one time or to using impure, adulterated material.

Since most of the complications and adverse reactions associated with silicone injections occurred because the compound was utilized incorrectly by inexperienced or unqualified professionals, the FDA in the United States placed this treatment technique under stringent restrictions back in 1965. Currently, silicone fluid still is being investigated under the "new drug" regulations of the United States government, whereby research and testing on human patients is limited to a small number of treatment centers.

As a matter of fact, under these rules, there are very few officially licensed physicians in the entire nation who are legally permitted to administer silicone injections. Seven of them have offices in New York City. These dozen dermatologists and plastic surgeons are the only ones who I would count on to inject bona fide silicone and to do the job right. So, if you are interested in obtaining this type of treatment for yourself, consult one of these highly skilled silicone specialists. Write to the FDA or ask your doctor for the names of physicians who are licensed silicone researchers in your geographical area.

What Silicone Is and How It Works

The proper chemical name of silicone is dimethylpolysiloxane. It is a concoction that belongs to a class of polymers made up of silicon, oxygen, and a bevy of organic materials. Manufactured and distributed in the United States *only* by the Dow-Corning Corporation, medical-grade silicone comes in a variety of physical forms.

Besides the highly purified liquid that is injectable, there are silicone foams, resins, sponges, and rubbers. As previously mentioned, the vulcanized rubber form of silicone is marketed as silastic, which can be safely and effectively implanted surgically to build up depressed, inadequate, or malformed chins, ears, noses, and breasts.

Silicone fluid—which is used for facial treatment

to fill in, plump up, eliminate, or improve unflattering lines, wrinkles, and sunken areas—has the distinct therapeutic advantage over the sponge and solid silicone implants of being injectable in very tiny volumes. The fact that significant cosmetic corrections can be achieved by having a series of shots in a doctor's office without having to undergo a surgical procedure makes this type of silicone treatment especially attractive. The simplicity and ease of delivery appeals to patients and doctors alike.

Unlike Zyderm-collagen, liquid silicone is injected *under* the skin rather than *into* its multiple layers. The placement of small amounts of silicone fluid beneath the skin stimulates the body's own fibrous tissue to surround each droplet of silicone fluid and hold it in place. Because the body identifies silicone as a foreign substance, it is not absorbed the same way Zyderm-collagen is, but remains permanently in a liquid state encapsulated within the body tissues as a multicystic fibrous mass.

In effect, pockets of encapsulated fat form around the tiny injected drops of silicone fluid. The silicone mass that is created fills in the empty spaces left by the missing body tissue, pushing out and propping up the drooping facial surface. Lines, wrinkles, and depressions disappear; sunken cheeks and contours are filled out and restored; and the skin is made firmer and smoother. The result: the face appears younger-looking and more attractive.

The key to the success of liquid silicone treatment is knowing exactly how much fluid to inject and exactly where to place it. Precision is of utmost importance, There is little room for error. Because the silicone fluid is not absorbed the way Zyderm-collagen is but stays put under the skin, any over-correction with too large an injection dose results in permanent bumps and distortion. That is why skilled, qualified physicians—the licensed researchers—are the only ones you should consult if you want to have this type of treatment.

These doctors know precisely how much sili-cone to use in each injection, how many injections are required, and how to space them to achieve optimal results. They also have the technical expertise to ad-minister the injections properly to prevent the migra-tion of silicone to other parts of your body.

A crucial step often involves the use of a hand-held vibrating machine, which the attending doctor applies to the treatment site for several minutes after each shot to evenly disperse the silicone fluid so that lumps, bumps, or localized cysts don't occur. Make certain that this is done to ensure best cosmetic results and prevent postinjection drifting of the silicone liquid.

Getting Silicone Injections

If you think silicone injections can correct your facial imperfections, do not consult anyone except one of the licensed silicone researchers. He will tell you whether this treatment is right for you and prescribe the appropriate injection regimen.

Bear in mind that, because silicone works best when administered in minute quantities, it can take up to ten sessions of silicone injections to fill out a minor wrinkle or small scar. Major imperfections require more extensive therapy over an extended time period.

It cannot be overemphasized that unless the proper scheduling of dosage amounts and intervals is strictly followed, untoward results—such as unsightly and potentially carcinogenic granuloma-like formations, localized swelling, and drifting—can occur. Any well-intentioned attempts to speed up the treatment by boosting the injection doses or shortening the intervals between them are ill-advised.

The cost of each silicone injection is less than for Zyderm-collagen, but you will probably need more shots of silicone to correct the same imperfection than would be necessary with Zyderm-collagen. Consequently, the costs of both types of treatment—Zyderm-collagen and silicone—work out to be about the same. You will pay less for each silicone injection but require more of them to achieve optimal correction of a particular defect.

Fees for correcting minimal wrinkles or scars with silicone shots run between $500 and $700. Total costs for silicone therapy to improve deep maximal scars or widespread wrinkles range between $2000 and $3000.

Silicone injections can be repeated at weekly intervals until the desired level of correction is achieved. Before each shot, the treatment area is scrubbed thoroughly with an antiseptic soap and then painted with a numbing solution of benzalkonium chloride.

To penetrate deep beneath the skin surface, the injection is delivered through a needle that is slightly thicker than the 30-gauge type used for Zyderm-collagen fluid, but still fine enough not to leave a lasting trace.

Following the silicone treatment, postinjection pain or discomfort is exceedingly rare. Swelling, too, is only minimal.

The improvement immediately visible after the silicone shot usually remains as is. There is very little dissipation of the implanted volume or loss of correction through absorption of the fluid. In fact, as the accumulated dosages of silicone build up, even the tiny volume losses that sometimes occur in the early stages of treatment diminish.

Corrections generally are long-lasting and permanent. Occasionally, some booster shots may be required at intervals several months apart to maintain or restore optimal correction.

As with Zyderm-collagen therapy, silicone injections work better on grosser defects. Fine lines and wrinkles are harder to correct, although shots of silicone can render noticeable—and in some cases, even remarkable—improvements on most varieties of facial imperfections.

However, it is important to note that deep lines around the lips are especially difficult to correct using silicone. In a tricky undertaking, the doctor must first undercut the lines to get underneath the defect before injecting the silicone fluid into the area. A similar technique is called for to improve "ice pick" acne scars, which can become exaggerated as a result of silicone therapy. Zyderm-collagen shots probably are a better bet for minimizing this type of acne scar, since they require less skill to administer and there is more room for error.

An important consideration in deciding whether to undergo silicone injections is that you can count on a prognosis of long-term safety and absence of negative reactions with silicone. Its track record as a safe, effective performer is both tested and assured.

Because silicone is inert, there is minimal risk of adverse tissue response, allergy development, and local inflammation. This is borne out by a protracted period of clinical experience, observation, and evaluation of silicone-injected patients. During the past twenty years, there never has been any incidence of allergic response, implant rejection, sensitization, or other health-harming consequences as a result of silicone-injection therapy administered by a physician licensed to use silicone.

Another salient fact: There never has been a malpractice suit against one of the licensed silicone re-searchers. Any problems or legal actions associated with silicone therapy in the past involved physicians or other practitioners who obtained impure silicone illegally and/or used liquid silicone improperly.

Unlike Zyderm-collagen, which won approval by the FDA in 1981 as a safe medical device, silicone fluid probably never will receive official government endorsement as a skin treatment, despite its long his-tory of safe, effective use. This is because its manu-facturer is not pressing for it. The Dow-Corning Corporation voluntarily withdrew its application for FDA approval of the sale of liquid silicone for skin treatment in 1975.

Still, silicone injections are an excellent therapeu-tic choice for correcting most major and minor facial imperfections. Lines, wrinkles, deep smile creases, frown furrows, sunken areas, depressed contours, and certain scars can be significantly improved without surgery, pain, or risk.

3 PUFFING OUT

If you wish you could make your unflattering wrinkles, scars, and craggy lines disappear but are afraid to try collagen or silicone, there is a third alternative you may want to consider. It is fibrin foam.

Interestingly enough, fibrin foam was the first nonsurgical treatment developed for wrinkles. Involving only a series of injections of a substance that is concocted from the patient's own blood, the therapy is both easy to take and easily tolerated. It is also extremely safe.

Hundreds of patients who have received fibrin-foam shots have been followed closely for periods of up to seventeen years with no signs of keloids (thick, fibrous scars), thickening of the treated areas, or any type of tumor reaction. In fact, there never has been an adverse reaction from this type of therapeutic procedure, which has been administered thousands of times.

Cosmetic results, too, are good. Injections of fibrin foam ultimately achieve solid improvements in an overwhelming proportion of patients. Wrinkles are puffed up and depressed scars filled out in more than 80 percent of the patients treated. And, as a bonus, unattractive lines are noticeably softened in 75 percent of the cases.

The shots, which can be administered in a doctor's office, require only a local anesthetic and are not painful, traumatic, or disfiguring. Causing minimal discomfort and necessitating no recovery regimen, fibrin-foam therapy is easy on the patient.

Although affordable, fibrin foam is not cheap, however. Because the substance is custom-made for each individual patient, laboratory fees are high. Charges for a batch of fibrin foam run in the range of $500 or more; but the substance keeps forever under refrigeration and can be drawn on indefinitely for further treatment and future maintenance. As a result, the initial expense may be higher for fibrin foam than for collagen or silicone, but in the long run treatment with fibrin foam may work out to be as reasonable as, or even cheaper than, the other two.

Fibrin foam was used frequently for cosmetic therapy about twenty years ago, before the medical profession became aware of the dangers of contracting hepatitis from using blood drawn from donors. At that time, the fibrin foam that was injected to correct facial defects was whipped up from so-called pool blood. Consequently, cases of hepatitis associated with the wrinkle treatment were not uncommon. Because hepatitis became a frequent side effect of fibrin-foam injections, this type of cosmetic therapy fell out of favor about ten years ago and was administered hardly at all.

Now that fibrin foam is specially prepared for each patient from her or his own blood, the risk of hepatitis is no longer a factor or consideration. This type of treatment is once more a viable alternative for minimizing or eliminating unsightly wrinkles and depressed scars.

Fibrin foam has many advantages. The fact that it is a natural injectable substance compatible with one's own body is a big plus. The chances of developing an allergic reaction are negligible. This means you do not have to have a preliminary skin test before undergoing fibrin-foam treatments. Another big plus for fibrin foam is that it is not photosensitizing. You can go out in the sun immediately after having a treatment and be unaffected. A further advantage is that you cannot come away from the therapy looking worse. Because fibrin foam is readily absorbed into your body tissue, excess quantities eventually disappear. In other words, the therapist can't make a mistake by injecting too much, an advantage fibrin foam shares with collagen over silicone.

Unlike collagen, which takes effect very quickly, fibrin foam is slow to work, which may be regarded as a disadvantage. Cosmetic therapy with fibrin foam requires patience from the patient.

Like silicone therapy, fibrin-foam treatment takes considerable time and necessitates many visits to the doctor before improvements are rendered. If you are looking for immediate gratification and quick results, this type of cosmetic therapy is not for you. Opt for collagen shots instead.

With collagen, which works very rapidly, you see results almost immediately—enabling you to judge whether the treatments are effective and stop them if they are not. This is not the case with fibrin foam. You cannot determine the efficacy of fibrin-foam injections while the treatment is in progress. Because of fibrin foam's delayed effect, you cannot be sure if it is really doing any good at all. You can go for many fibrin-foam injections without visible results, and it is possible you will never see any at all. In other words, you have to stick with the therapy, even if you do not notice any change, and hope for the best.

What Fibrin Foam Is and How It Is Made

Fibrin is a blood substance used medically in a gel foam to promote coagulation during surgery. The particular fibrin substance that is formulated for cosmetic facial treatment—fibrin foam—is made especially for each individual patient prior to initiating the injection therapy.

A test tube full of blood is taken from the patient

and shipped off to the laboratory. There the fibrin is extracted by spinning the blood and removing the red blood cells, which are discarded. Then technicians painstakingly adjust the pH of the serum that is left by adding minuscule quantities of various saline solutions in stages until the right balance is achieved. The resulting white pasty powder is the essence of fibrin foam. A potent biological substance, it is combined with either one of two anesthetics—Xylocaine or novocaine—for painless injection.

Another, much cheaper, method of making a type of fibrin foam for cosmetic therapy was developed by a Washington, D.C., physician. Called the GAP Method (because it fills the "gap"), it involves much less laboratory work. The extracted serum from the patient's blood simply is added to a patented secret formula.

The formula consists of a sterilized gel foam, like that used in surgery, in combination with delta amino levulinic acid, a fibrin stabilizer. The gel foam substitutes for the much more expensive pH-adjusted fibrin foam. Because of the presence of delta amino levulinic acid, which can be fatal in large doses, the GAP-method version of fibrin foam is considered by the FDA to be a drug that requires government approval—which it has not yet secured—for widespread use and distribution.

In addition to the two basic methods of preparing fibrin foam, there are variations in the way the substance is applied therapeutically. Some doctors contend that fibrin foam works better when it is activated by freshly drawn serum. Consequently, to make it more effective, many therapists take a small amount of blood from the patient at the start of each treatment visit, spin the extracted fluid in a special vessel to remove the red blood cells, and then add the fresh serum to the patient's ready stock of fibrin foam before injecting it.

Other fibrin-foam therapists contend that adding small bits of the patient's skin to the fibrin foam enhances the filling-out process. To do this, they remove a minuscule amount of flesh from the patient's thigh or bottom and emulsify it in a blender. The fragments are then mixed into the fibrin foam. The doctors who regularly follow this regimen insist that the added bulk works better to fill in wrinkles and scars and has the further advantage of being a natural substance from the patient's own body.

How Fibrin Foam Works

Fibrin foam is injected *under* the skin rather than *into* it. The procedure involves a tricky technique that is crucial to its success.

The wrinkle or scar being treated first must be undermined before it can be corrected. To do this, the doctor must carefully separate the wrinkle or scar from the underlying skin by cutting away the epidermis, or topmost skin layer, from the dermis, or supporting layer, and shooting the fibrin foam underneath the epidermis. The procedure is a combination of separation and injection that requires precision and artistry for best results.

Fibrin foam fills out and builds up unsightly depressions on your face by becoming part of the support system beneath the surface. Absorbed into the dermal layer below, fibrin foam replaces deficient collagen and props up sags and crags, making wrinkles, scars, and lines disappear.

The optimal amount of fibrin foam to be injected is that which is necessary to achieve 110 percent correction, or just enough to build up the wrinkle, or puff out the scar, slightly above the level of surrounding skin. Since fibrin foam is readily absorbed, it is impossible to have too much injected. If too little is injected to produce the desired correction, the procedure may be repeated at two-month intervals until results are satisfactory.

Obtaining Fibrin-Foam Therapy

Seek out a dermatologist who frequently gives fibrinfoam shots and get his opinion as to whether this therapy is right for you. He will probably show you one or more medical articles on the subject before initiating the treatments. If he does not, ask to see some reference material to familiarize yourself with the therapy in order to know what to expect.

At the outset of each treatment visit, the wrinkle or scar to be corrected is outlined with a skin-marking pencil. Then novocaine is injected beneath the area with a fine 26-gauge needle.

Next the needle hole is enlarged by shooting some additional novocaine through a thicker, 20-gauge needle. This makes way for a diamond-shaped instrument to be inserted through the second novocaine hole.

A specially designed medical tool called the undercutting blade, with cutting edges on all four sides, is manipulated back and forth horizontally to undermine the wrinkle or scar and create a pocket for the fibrin foam. Finally, the fibrin foam itself is shot into the same hole, which is closed up afterward by the chemical action of a droplet of flexible collodion, a medical glue.

The degree of success that is ultimately achieved from fibrin-foam therapy depends to a large extent on the technical skill of the treatment specialist and how he performs the crucial undermining step. If he undermines the wrinkle or scar at too deep a level, the unsightly defect merely will be raised up and appear unchanged. If he cuts at too shallow a level, he may penetrate the skin surface, causing the fibrin foam to leak out and be lost. For best results, the wrinkle or scar must be undermined at just the right level for the fibrin foam to puff up and smooth out the unflattering depression on the facial surface above. That is why a dermatologist experienced with fibrin-foam therapy is your best bet if you decide you want to undertake this type of cosmetic treatment.

Your body will not reject fibrin foam. Because it is basically compatible with your system, tissue expulsion never occurs and there is no possibility of your having an allergic reaction. All traces of fibrin foam eventually disappear within your body as the substance is absorbed into the surrounding tissues and becomes part of the collagen network, which bolsters and supports the skin.

The only problems ever reported as a consequence of fibrin-foam therapy—bacterial infections—have nothing to do with the injected substance itself but are caused by the needle punctures. Such infections, which can develop after any type of injection or shot, are a minimal risk and occur in less than half of one percent of the total number of treatments administered. But there are several important drawbacks to fibrin foam. It is not readily available because it is made from an individual's own blood, is slow to work, and requires many treatments. The results are not dramatic, and it is not always effective.

4 SPEEDING UP

If you are displeased with yourself because the tone and texture of your skin are not what they once were, don't despair. There are revolutionary medicines and new do-it-yourself techniques and products available to help you rejuvenate and revitalize your aging skin.

The things we are talking about are not risky, harmful, or painful. They entail minimal expense, no serious side effects, and hardly any effort. Safe and effective, these preparations and practices produce significant results fairly quickly. Your skin will appear noticeably smoother and sport a better blush of color. You will look more youthful and healthier, too.

These latest developments in skin care improve your appearance by affecting the topmost tier of the epidermis—the stratum corneum. Skin gets blotchy and rough and loses its youthful glow when this top layer of cells is not replaced as often as needed. Old, dead cells tend to accumulate on the skin surface, giving it an uneven tone and texture.

This happens as you get older because the reproduction rate of skin cells slows down. Fresh, moist cells are not produced rapidly enough to replenish the dried-out cells on the surface to maintain a soft, smooth, and rosy complexion.

There are several ways to speed up the cell turnover time for the stratum corneum that can soften and smooth your skin and restore its youthful blush. The effect can be achieved by medication—topical and oral—or by physical means. Either is effective alone but both work especially well in synergistic combination.

Anti-Aging Medication

As far as the medications are concerned, there is a patented formula you apply to your skin that is truly anti-aging. Available by prescription, it can be used not only to reverse the ravaged appearance of elderly skin but also to prevent skin from ever getting old-looking.

Called Retin-A, this FDA-approved topical drug was developed by its manufacturer, Johnson & Johnson, as an acne medicine. Later found to be equally effective for improving the appearance of aged skin, Retin-A has been used successfully for skin treatment and maintenance. It is not FDA-approved for anti-aging treatments.

Retin-A is one of many innovative medications derived from Vitamin-A acid, or retinoic acid, a toxic substance which when targeted to the skin has a beneficial effect. Interestingly enough, this medication, when taken orally or applied topically, speeds up cell production and development in the underlying layers of skin, which works to cure acne and destroy premalignant conditions.

The reason Retin-A also improves the quality of elderly skin is that the condition of older skin resembles that of a premalignancy. The physical characteristics of both are virtually identical.

Applications of Retin-A increase both the number and size of skin cells on the stratum corneum, the visible surface of the skin. Observed under a microscope, the pattern produced by the newly formed skin cells is very much like that of a newborn baby's. In effect, Retin-A can turn back the clock for skin and restore it to a more youthful condition. Put another way, Retin-A has a truly miraculous effect on postpubescent skin that is acne-ridden or otherwise damaged from age or excessive sun exposure. Such skin is transformed to its prepubescent state of rosy softness and smoothness.

Orally administered versions of Vitamin-A acid —retinoids—also are prescribed mostly to treat acne but work equally well in low doses to reverse the damaged appearance of elderly skin. In fact, within the next five years, it is expected that retinoids will be adapted for widespread use as the first oral anti-aging prophylactic. One major drawback is that they can cause birth defects in pregnant women. Consult your physician.

What Retin-A Is and How It Works

Retin-A is a patented Vitamin-A compound that is available by prescription in gel, cream, and liquid forms. The gel is the mildest concentration. The liquid is the most potent.

When applied to the skin, Retin-A kicks up the cell turnover on the stratum corneum by stimulating mitotic activity in the basal layer below. New cells are produced more rapidly and divide at an accelerated rate, gradually moving in a mass toward the surface. The upward migration of the new cells helps to clear the visible surface of unsightly oily accumulations, crusty brown spots, whiteheads, and dead cells by pushing up the oil cups around the skin glands, dislodging the contents, and flushing them away.

Needless to say, the medication is somewhat irritating, even in its weakest form, but most patients find it tolerable. Retin-A also is drying since it removes significant amounts of oil from the skin surface. You can compensate for this by applying a moisturizing emollient to replenish the lost oil.

Retin-A clears the complexion of unattractive pimples, discolorations, and other surface irregularities. As a matter of fact, it is because acne patients observed that the normal skin adjacent to acne-ridden areas looked noticeably better that Retin-A began to be used for skin revitalization and care.

You can dilute Retin-A with Nivea, or any other emollient lotion or cream, on a one-to-one basis and use the mixture regularly as an anti-aging moisturizer to prevent your skin from becoming rough, blotchy, and drab-colored. The approximate cost of this highly beneficial beauty aid is a mere $7 for a six-week supply, which is considerably cheaper than most of the over-the-counter moisturizers you can buy. People between the ages of thirty and forty would be well advised to start applying a Retin-A-based moisturizer at least once a day as a maintenance regimen.

Be aware, however, that Retin-A, even when diluted, causes photosensitization in 50 percent of its users. So do not apply it before going to the beach or out into the sun. Direct exposure to sunlight could make the treated areas redden intensely or could trigger a sensitivity reaction.

Retin-A erases the damage wrought on skin by excessive exposure to the sun—brown spots, leathery toughness, and unattractive ruddiness. Retin-A also is excellent for treating Darier's disease, which causes a particular premature aging in young people that is characterized by gross thickening of the skin. In addition, Retin-A is sometimes prescribed as a successful antidote for another skin-aging affliction, lichen-planus disease, which produces a slowing down of the cell turnover time in the stratum corneum. Retin-A treats both diseases by accelerating the production rate and migration of skin cells, thus restoring a healthy, young-looking skin surface.

Using Retin-A

You can get a prescription to purchase Retin-A from any doctor. Your best bet, however, is to consult a dermatologist who is familiar with this innovative medication to see if it is right for your skin.

Once you are ready to use this topical drug, embark on a one-month program. Have a close-up photograph taken of yourself. Start out by applying Retin-A gel, cream, or liquid full strength to your skin once a day. It may be irritating for the first week. If you find you can tolerate the medication this way, step up your applications to twice a day for the next three weeks. After the initial month is over, take another photograph and compare the two of them. You should observe a marked improvement in your appearance. If you are satisfied with what you see, proceed by using Retin-A once a day on a permanent basis as an anti-aging cream.

If you find you cannot tolerate Retin-A full

strength because it is too drying or irritating, dilute it with Nivea cream or Pond's Cold Cream in equal portions and follow the same regimen outlined above. And, if the diluted version of Retin-A still is too harsh on your skin, try substituting for the Nivea or Pond's, as a dilutant, Cortaid, an excellent anti-inflammatory cream you can buy over-the-counter without a prescription. Follow the same initial month-long regimen. If you get satisfactory results, cut back to applying the same mixture once a day for maintenance of young-looking skin.

When using Retin-A, start with the weakest strength. Avoid the sun and be prepared for some irritation. Here is a step-by-step program for using Retin-A:

1. Wash face for about three minutes with cool water using an oily-type soap like Dove, Tone, or Oilatum. Do not over-scrub.

2. The first week, take a small amount of Retin-A gel (the weakest formulation of this medication). If necessary, mix it one-to-one with Pond's Cold Cream or Nivea cream, and rub gently onto entire area of aging skin, allowing the medication to penetrate for two or three minutes. Apply Retin-A before makeup in the morning and again, if tolerable, at

night. Use daily if possible; but if your skin becomes irritated, alternate days or apply every third day.

3. The second week, increase the proportions of Retin-A to two-thirds Retin-A and one-third cold cream.

4. The third and fourth week, use Retin-A alone.

5. Check with your doctor for instructions on how to use Retin-A on a permanent basis as an anti-aging cream.

For maximum results, increase the strength of Retin-A by changing from gel to cream, then cream to liquid, month by month, although you do not have to go to the most potent form of Retin-A to obtain good results. You can stay at the strength that you find comfortable. If you change from the milder gel to the stronger cream or liquid, begin by diluting with cold cream as before to avoid severe irritation. Stop using this medication the day before you plan to go out in strong sun.

What Retinoids Are and How They Work

Retinoids are potent prescription drugs that contain Vitamin-A in its acid form as their principal active ingredient. Taken orally to cure acne, these medications have certain side effects and should be used with caution.

Retinoids can be toxic. They raise the fat content of blood to levels that can trigger heart attacks in people prone to cardiovascular disease. They can cause birth defects. Be aware, too, that retinoids also produce an uncomfortable dryness of the lips and eyes.

But these oral medications have some beneficial side effects as well. Because of the way they interact with particular mucous cells, retinoids prevent cancers from developing in the mouth, bladder, and lungs.

While highly effective for treating acne, retinoids still are in the experimental stage as far as anti-aging applications are concerned. Nevertheless, the biology of skin and the chemical makeup of the drugs suggest that this group of medications is highly promising for eventual adaptation to reverse or prevent unattractive aging of the skin.

Accutane, like other retinoids, works to improve acne-ridden skin and blotchy, uneven complexions by internally stimulating the generation of new skin cells to replace the damaged stratum corneum. The unattractive skin surface is shed and a new one is formed with a greater quantity of larger cells, which make your skin look younger. You see a difference in your skin within a week's time. Your complexion has a smoother, younger look. Retinoids act similarly to steroid hormones in that they make skin feel soft and give it a nice blush. For anti-aging treatments, a lower dose than for acne is recommended.

Epidermabrasion

The key to maintaining a healthy, young-looking complexion is keeping up the frequent and steady cell turnover in the stratum corneum, or topmost skin layer. As explained above, applying certain chemicals topically or taking them by mouth accelerates the turnover time of cells on the skin surface, making skin look better.

But the same effect can be achieved by do-it-yourself mechanical stimulation. In other words, there is a way you can handle and care for your skin that makes it smoother, softer, clearer, and rosier. You can rid your complexion of unsightly blotches, raised brown spots, crusty accumulations, white-heads, small pimples, and other surface irregularities. All you have to do is utilize the proper technique in everyday cleansing.

The technique is called epidermabrasion, which is a fancy word for aggressively rubbing your skin while washing it with soap and water. Epiderma-brasion works directly on the stratum corneum by scraping off dry, dead cells, excess oils, discolored buildups, and other debris. Rubbing the skin's surface stimulates the growth of new cells underneath. The abrasive action also increases blood flow within the skin cells. The improved circulation gives your complexion a healthy glow.

Even if you have dry skin, you still can epiabrade without excessively drying out your skin. Use a moisturizing lotion instead of soap and water as a lubricant and epiabrade your face at least once a day.

The most effective epiabrading tool is the readily available Buf-Puf. Sold in drugstores and supermarkets everywhere, this polyester, spongelike web has many advantages. Besides being moderately priced, it is easy to handle and to clean, as well as reusable and very durable. You can control the intensity of epidermabrasion by how much pressure you exert on the Buf-Puf and how rapidly you move it across your skin. You can build up your tolerance for epidermabrasion by gradually increasing pressure and speed. For optimal effect, epiabrade as vigorously and often as you can withstand without irritating your skin.

Daily epidermabrasion definitely improves the look and feel of the stratum corneum. It becomes softer and smoother and develops a more even tone and texture. Epidermabrasion can supplement regular use of Retin-A to maintain a healthy-looking skin surface.

If your skin is unusually tender and you find the Buf-Puf too abrasive, you can epiabrade with a soft washcloth and still get good results. Sea sponges and loofahs tend to be harsher and more expensive than the Buf-Puf but are effective epiabrading tools, nevertheless. Some people prefer them because they are made of natural fibers even though they are less flexible and harder to clean than the synthetic Buf-Puf.

Here is an easy-to-follow program for epidermabrasion. Follow this regimen three to seven days a week, depending on your skin's level of irritation:

1. Using a mild soap, wash face with cool water. For the first two weeks of this regimen, use a milder soap than you would ordinarily.

2. Leave face damp with a small residue of soap.

3. Using a Buf-Puf, a loofah, or a washcloth, epiabrade gently in circular motions. Start by doing this for two minutes in the morning and again at night, gradually increasing by one minute a week until you reach five minutes in the morning and five minutes at night.

4. After epiabrading, rinse face and apply a mild moisturizer.

5. Now apply makeup if desired.

If irritation occurs at any time, discontinue for a while; resume when irritation subsides, but for a decreased time. You will get less irritation in the summer than in the winter.

A-Hydroxy-Acid Moisturizers

Most moisturizing lotions have only a temporary effect on the existing stratum corneum. They contain water to hydrate it and emollients to smooth it. Such moisturizers do not change the permanent condition of the stratum corneum by affecting the formation of the critical skin layer itself. However, there are some moisturizing products with certain ingredients that do work to trigger the growth of a new, healthier stratum corneum to replace the damaged or old-looking one.

These moisturizers contain one or more of the alpha-hydroxy, or A-hydroxy, acids, a large group of organic compounds, many of which occur naturally in foods. Common A-hydroxy acids that are incorporated in cosmetic products include citric acid (which is found in citrus fruits), malic acid (present in apples), lactic acid (in sour milk), quinic acid (in apples and other fruits), and tartaric acid (in grape wine and fruits).

Cosmetic products with A-hydroxy acids are therapeutically beneficial to aged or sun-damaged skin that is marred with unattractive brown spots and surface irregularities. The organic acids act to refurbish the stratum corneum by promoting the discarding of the existing surface and its replacement with a fresh one populated by plump, moist cells. In fact, A-hydroxy acids really do not function as moisturizers. By causing a resurfacing of the skin, they obviate the need for a moisturizer.

Still, the vast majority of products with A-hydroxy acids are labeled moisturizers. One such product is Lacticare. Widely available over-the-counter in pharmacies and department stores, this reasonably priced product, which contains lactic acid, helps dry, elderly skin regain its dewy softness.

Here is a daily regimen for using A-hydroxy acid moisturizers to keep your skin looking young. Follow this procedure two or three times a day, more frequently in winter than in summer:

1. Wash face with soap and warm water for two to four minutes, using a pH-balanced soap, such as Dove, to maintain the acidity of skin. Do not use Ivory with this regimen, because it is too alkaline. Be sure to remove all traces of soap, but leave a small residue of water on face.
2. Dab an amount the size of a quarter of A-hydroxy acid moisturizer on each side of your face and rub it vigorously into the skin.
3. Now apply makeup, if desired.

All A-hydroxy acids work the same way. Try the cheapest available brand of moisturizer first, but if it does not work for you within two weeks, change to a different one. If irritation occurs, discontinue for several days and then start again. You may not experience irritation the second time around. Every four to six weeks, switch brands of A-hydroxy acid moisturizers. Your skin can build up a tolerance to the medication, making it less effective.

5 GROWING NEW SKIN

If you have indulged in too much sun and feel self-conscious about your brown-blotched, crepe-textured, or otherwise prematurely old-looking skin, there is a surefire way to restore your youthful good looks that doesn't require any surgery or even a shot. It is another revolutionary do-it-yourself prescription medicine you can buy and dab on that will literally help grow attractive, healthy new skin.

Like Retin-A, it is safe and highly effective for revitalizing aged or sun-damaged skin that is not too wrinkled. This FDA-approved topical medication is called Efudex and is manufactured by Hoffmann–La Roche. Available in cream and liquid form, it is excellent for treating—and replacing—skin that is thin, discolored, or leathery from the natural wear and tear of aging or from excessive exposure to the sun. A virtual fountain of youth, Efudex also can be relied on for once-a-week use to prevent skin from ever growing old.

Efudex can be smeared or swabbed onto your face, on the backs of your hands, or anywhere on your body to make your skin appear younger and healthier. It really works wonders on skin that looks old even though it is relatively unwrinkled. For people who apply Efudex twice a day to grow new skin, the success rate is a whopping 93 percent. You see a dramatic transformation after three months. The new skin that appears is smoother, softer, and noticeably younger-looking.

Considering the results you get, Efudex is a real bargain. The amount needed to treat your entire face will set you back betwen $20 and $100, depending on the quantity you use. When used prophylactically, Efudex costs hardly anything.

Keep in mind, however, that until you grow your new skin layer, you can look like a mess for quite some time and experience some discomfort. Your skin will become red and blistery and feel sore. People with light eyes usually have a more severe reaction than others. Moreover, the drug can be unpredictable in terms of how long it takes to achieve results.

Remember, too, that Efudex is photosensitizing. Be sure to avoid the sun or cover treated areas with sunscreen whenever Efudex is used.

What Efudex Is and How It Works

Efudex is a patented medicine that was developed to treat cancers internally. While still used for that purpose, the formula—which contains as its basic active ingredient the fluorinated compound 5-fluorouracil—has been adapted for topical use to treat certain skin cancers and to refurbish aged and sun-damaged skin.

Efudex Cream contains 5 percent fluorouracil in a vanishing-cream base that consists of white petrolatum plus alcohol, moisturizing propylene glycol, and some paraben preservatives. Efudex Solution contains 2 to 5 percent fluorouracil compounded with moisturizing propylene glycol and paraben preservatives. Be advised that propylene glycol can be irritating to sensitive skin and that paraben preservatives sometimes precipitate sensitivity reactions in the allergy-prone.

Efudex Cream is rubbed into your skin; Efudex Solution is swabbed onto it. Both are equally effective for treating damaged-looking skin, but the cream usually is preferred for prophylactic use to prevent aging.

The reason Efudex works so well to reverse the ravaged appearance of aged and sun-damaged skin is that such skin has atypical cells which exhibit a growth pattern markedly similar to that of cancerous cells and unlike that of healthy young skin.

Healthy young skin constantly refreshes itself with new cells. Produced in batches at regular intervals in the bottommost skin layers, the new cells travel together as a group toward the surface. This upward migration usually takes about two weeks. In the course of the journey, the cells lose moisture. Dried-up cells get sloughed off at the top but are immediately replaced with fresh moist ones in a never-ending cycle.

Aged and sun-damaged skin cells do not develop and grow the same way as healthy young cells. They reproduce erratically. Instead of traveling upward together in a pack, their new skin cells migrate helter-skelter in all directions and lose their cohesiveness. They move away from each other in random fashion. All this uncoordinated movement within the skin layers creates thin areas, vascular eruptions, and crusty patches on the visible surface above.

Unlike collagen and silicone, which change the appearance of the skin surface by affecting the underlying dermal layer, Efudex, like Retin-A, works directly on the epidermis. It treats the surface by selectively destroying the atypical cells that are responsible for the thinness, roughness, and blotchiness that characterize old or sun-damaged skin.

Efudex's basic ingredient—the fluorinated compound 5-fluorouracil—blocks the atypical cells' synthesis of DNA and RNA, which are essential for cell division and growth. The resulting DNA and RNA deprivation is suspected of causing thymine deficiency, which promotes the death of the abnormal cells.

Interestingly enough, Efudex affects only abnormal cells—those of aged or sun-damaged skin. It is not absorbed by healthy skin cells or by any other part of your body system. Moreover, the more atypical a cell is, the more it is affected by the drug. It is because Efudex is selectively picked up by atypical cells, which eventually produce unflattering skin conditions, that the medication can be used prophylactically to prevent visible flaws.

Using Efudex

You can obtain a prescription for Efudex from any licensed physician here in the United States or buy it over-the-counter in Europe, where it is widely available. Nevertheless, your best bet is to consult a dermatologist or an internist who is familiar with the medication to make certain that this particular therapeutic drug is appropriate for you and your skin. Because systemic absorption of Efudex is insignificant, this topical medication generally is considered safe for most people, but is not recommended for use by pregnant women.

To replace old-looking or sun-damaged skin, apply Efudex Cream or Efudex Solution twice a day for a period of two to four weeks. Be sure to completely cover all the areas you want to treat. You probably will not notice any change in your appearance during the first two weeks.

In the third week, you will see your skin suddenly start to turn red. The redness will become more vivid, itch and hurt, and then ulcerate and ooze. The blisters will vary in severity because of the uneven distribution of sun-damaged skin. But even moderately sun-damaged skin has a significant reaction.

Once your skin erupts, stop applying the medication. At this point, start to apply cool compresses to your skin, which will look beet-red and be covered with weeping sores. The compresses will help to make you more comfortable and alleviate the inflammation and swelling. Or, if you prefer, rub in some cortisone cream, which is available without a prescription, to reduce the swelling. In acute cases, you might want to ask your physician for a prescription for cortisone to be taken orally. During this stage, you must scrupulously avoid the sun to prevent the red pigmentation from baking into your skin.

You can expect the redness to fade away gradually over the following few weeks. In the meantime, you can cover the inflammation with makeup. The lesions on your skin will take another month or two to heal and disappear.

Continue using the cortisone cream for two or three weeks. Then stop applying it and see what happens. The roughness, thinness, and leathery texture should be gone. Your skin should be baby soft and smooth. You probably will look ten years younger and may feel rejuvenated as well.

There are ways to speed up the drug's effect on your skin, but do not attempt such steps on your face. If you want to obtain a quicker reaction on the backs of your hands, for example, apply Efudex and then go out in the sun. Placing an occlusive dressing over the treated area also intensifies the reaction but is not recommended for your face.

Efudex generally produces excellent results without any untoward aftereffects. Occasionally, however, there is splotchy dark discoloration that may persist, but it is usually associated with sun exposure and occurs in less than 5 percent of Efudex users. In rare cases, there is keloidal scarring. To avoid this, anyone with any tendency toward this condition should try Efudex on the backs of her or his hands or on a small skin area before attempting to apply it to the face for intensive cosmetic therapy.

To use Efudex prophylactically to prevent your skin from aging, just take a small amount of the cream or solution once a week and rub it or swab it into your skin. You can cover the treated area with makeup. But be sure to apply a sunscreen, like PreSun 15, over the area at all times; and avoid direct exposure to sunlight.

Efudex is unpredictable, so be careful. Be sure to avoid the sun. Since this medicine irritates, do not begin using it if you have to look flawless in the near future.

Here is a step-by-step regimen to rejuvenate sun-damaged skin with Efudex:

1. Wash face with warm water for two to three minutes with a mildly drying soap like Ivory or Lifebuoy.
2. Twice a day for two to four weeks, or until skin becomes irritated, rub a small amount of Efudex, in cream or liquid form, into the affected areas.
3. Stop applying the medication as soon as the skin appears irritated and turns red. The onset of irritation may take anywhere from two to eight weeks.
4. Then apply cool compresses and/or cortisone cream to irritated areas two or three times a day. The irritation should subside in about two weeks, but may last six or eight weeks.

Sun makes this medicine work faster but also causes more irritation. If you use Efudex for three weeks and see nothing happening, try exposing the treated areas to a little sun.

After the initial treatment, Efudex should be used every six months to maintain younger-looking skin. As before, wash face with drying soap and apply medicine twice a day for three weeks, then discontinue even if there is no irritation.

6 CLEARING UP

If telltale aging signs—such as red spots, brown patches, fine lines, little crags, or a drab complexion—are getting you down, you can pick yourself up without spending a lot of time or money. There are some quick-acting, easy-to-take therapies and products available to help you look and feel younger and more attractive.

Red Spots

Little red spots, or broken blood vessels, that appear suddenly around your nose or elsewhere on your face can be removed without much fuss or bother for under $100. You have a choice of three methods for getting rid of these complexion-marring imperfections, which are technically dubbed "spider angiomas." All require a visit to a doctor, usually a dermatologist, for a treatment that lasts between twenty minutes and half an hour.

You can have red spots literally shocked off. This is done using a very fine needle made out of titanium that is mounted on an electric-powered instrument. In his or her office, the physician touches the needle to the blood vessel. The treatment is not painless. Like any electric shock, it produces an uncomfortable or painful sensation. Fortunately, the unpleasantness is brief and has its rewards. The current "fries" the blood vessel and destroys it, clearing your face of the annoying eyesore.

Be aware, however, that one treatment may not be enough to do the job. Most doctors are conservative in handling this power-driven needle, since it can produce a hole or depressed scar where the blood vessel existed if it is held in place too long. Therefore, the entire blood vessel may not be destroyed the first time around and a second treatment may be required to finish it off.

Another option is to have red spots removed by means of an Argon laser beam. Interestingly, outside the United States, in Europe and Israel, the use of laser machines for skin therapy and chronic care of the complexion is gaining widespread popularity.

A series of ten low-level laser-beam treatments is becoming the rage abroad as the poor man's alternative to an expensive face-lift. This laser therapy, which costs about $20 for each individual session, produces a sunburnlike irritation, which puffs out lines and wrinkles and boosts blood circulation. The result: skin appears smoother and sports a youthful blush. To keep the complexion looking this way, re-treatment is necessary every four months, or three times a year. This treatment can cause damage to eyes and skin and should be approached with extreme caution.

While chronic bombardment with low-level laser beams is probably successful in making people look younger and better, the long-term impact of this therapy on the health of the patient—particularly on the eyes—is unknown. Here in the United States, lasers for *this* use are not FDA-approved medical devices and few doctors have these costly machines at their disposal.

Nevertheless, where available, lasers can be harnessed effectively to erase red areas—unsightly port-wine stains of various sizes that mark some people at birth and blood-vessel eruptions that develop from excessive sun exposure or natural aging late in life. An experienced laser-beam therapist can carefully focus and target the rays at the unflattering red blotches and obliterate them. Be advised, however, that the long-term risks of such therapy still are not determined.

Red spots also can be removed by injection. The procedure, which can be done in a doctor's office, is completely safe and involves no risks. The physician shoots a saline solution directly into the visible blood vessel. The injection hurts only minimally and works rapidly to eliminate the eyesore by causing the blood vessel to burst and release the blood.

Brown Patches

Flat or raised brown patches, which appear on your forehead, cheeks, or upper lip as you get older, often are caused by excessive sun exposure. But they also develop in some women when there is an overabundance of estrogen in the body, as in pregnancy.

Flat brown blotches are not conducive to surgical removal because depressed scars are likely to result. Until recently, the treatment of choice for assured safety was Porcelana, or some variation of this mild, slow-acting over-the-counter product, like Esotérica and Nudit Gentle Skin Lightener with Sunscreen. These readily available commercial formulas all contain minuscule amounts of an effective bleaching agent—hydroquinone—and take a very long time to gradually fade out the unattractive discoloration.

Now, however, there's a revolutionary fast-acting combination of creams you can buy with a prescription for about $30. Applied daily, the creams work synergistically to rapidly erase the brown patches from your skin. Your complexion will be completely clear within three months. While the medication has a built-in sunscreen, it is best to avoid direct exposure to the sun during the treatment period.

The first cream—Eldoquin Forte—is smeared on in the morning after you wash your face but before you apply your makeup. It contains a potent concentration of hydroquinone for quick bleaching action.

The second cream, which is rubbed in around midday, is the highly effective Retin-A, a patented formula by Johnson & Johnson (see chapter 4). It is included to accelerate the skin-cell turnover time in order to bring the unwanted pigment rapidly to the surface.

The third cream, which is applied before bedtime, is a cortisone-based formula, designed to cut down the inflammatory reaction brought about by the irritating action of the two other creams. It works by precipitating a constriction of the blood vessels, which reduces swelling and redness and prevents the absorption of the medication itself into the bloodstream. These fast-acting creams work quickly and safely to fade out brown splotches that mar the skin on your face, hands, or body.

Another effective topical medication for erasing brown pigmentation is Neutrogena Melanex. It has a special base which is formulated to deliver the hydroquinone directly into the skin's pigment source, the hair-follicle cells beneath the surface.

While most people can tolerate this medication without suffering an allergic or sensitivity reaction, a few individuals sometimes find it irritating. If you experience some form of mild irritation, ask the pharmacist to make up the prescription substituting "Neutrogena Vehicle N Mild" (with less alcohol) to dilute the regular formula.

If you lack the patience to apply the fast-working creams and want to see immediate results, more radical remedies for ridding yourself of flat brown spots are available. You can have the coloration buzzed away with a brief electric treatment in a doctor's office for under $50. The therapist passes the electric current through an orange peel held against your face. Medical experts aren't sure exactly why this works, but the orange peel absorbs the discolored pigment, leaving your complexion clear. The therapy involves some minor discomfort.

Flat brown spots also can be burned off, scraped off, or frozen and then removed by a dermatologist or other qualified physician in a doctor's office. While these minor surgical procedures are not a big deal, certain aftereffects are possible. You could wind up with darker or lighter skin patches at the removal sites. Blacks are predisposed to developing white spots where something is excised. Getting rid of flat brown spots by any of these methods will cost between $100 and $500.

If you leave your flat brown spots alone, chances

are they eventually will become raised. This condition is called "seborrheic keratosis," and is responsive to three different types of therapy.

You can have the protruding defects cut away with a scalpel, in a minor surgical procedure that requires only a local anesthetic, like novocaine. A dermatologist or other medical doctor can do it in her or his office. Incisions can be sewn up less noticeably if you have a conveniently situated line or wrinkle to hide the stitches. Be aware, however, that you could end up with a depressed scar or white mark exactly the same size as whatever it is you are having removed.

Raised brown spots also can be burned off with an electric needle or an acid in a doctor's office. Both methods are equally effective for doing away with such imperfections. In either case, however, you may end up with a scar or white depression. Any of the above three removal procedures for raised brown spots range in cost from $100 to $500.

Electronic Facial

For a refreshing and rejuvenating experience, try an electronic facial. It is just the thing to make you look your best and feel more self-confident for a big occasion—a class reunion, a critical business meeting, or a family wedding.

Any dermatologist can do it for the price of an office visit, or between $30 and $100. It takes only fifteen minutes and involves minimal pain and discomfort.

You sit in a chair while the doctor uses a specially designed power instrument to pass an electric current gently over your face. The effect is that of a vigorous epidermabrasion.

The electric friction rubs off most of the existing stratum corneum, or covering layer of skin, along with small imperfections—tiny blood vessels and veins, developing sun-induced keratoses, or crusty brown patches, and other unsightly discolorations and irregularities—and stimulates more rapid production of fresh skin cells to replace the damaged surface. This causes a beneficial irritation that is characterized by a small amount of swelling and red-tinged coloration in the topmost tier of skin cells.

The barely detectable puffiness is just enough to push out fine lines and plump up small wrinkles, making them disappear completely or appear much less noticeable. The heightened redness gives the complexion a healthy glow similar to that produced by a slight sunburn.

As a result, you look better and younger for a couple of weeks. For best results, plan to have an electronic facial about five days to a week ahead of the momentous occasion.

7 PEELING OFF

If you cannot tolerate your own face because it is etched with fine lines and wrinkles around the mouth or tiny creases across the forehead—aging signs that collagen and silicone can do little to correct—there is a surefire remedy for doing away with those unflattering skin defects. The remedy is deep chemical peelings, a process that is neither quick to take effect nor easy to undergo, but one that really works wonders to eliminate those unwanted little imperfections that make you look years older than you either are or would like to appear.

Deep chemical peelings will set you back between $3000 and $5000. While slow to work and temporarily disfiguring, these treatments usually achieve dramatic results. You may look and feel awful for several weeks, but the ultimate improvement you see could make all the trouble, discomfort, and expense worthwhile.

Unfortunately, this type of treatment has received negative publicity because of irresponsible and improper applications. The fact is that deep chemical peelings fall into the category of facials, which, legally, anyone is allowed to give for cosmetic purposes. Nevertheless, since this particular facial involves the use of potent and irritating acid substances on skin surfaces, medical problems can and do occur.

That is why you would be wise to consult a qualified dermatologist who frequently does deep chemical peelings if you are interested in safely erasing minor lines and wrinkles. Get her or his opinion on whether this type of treatment is appropriate for you.

Be advised that deep chemical peelings work best on fair-skinned people. The darker your complexion, the less successful the treatments are likely to be. That is because blotchiness is more likely to develop on deeper-toned skin, and the demarcation line between treated and untreated areas also is apt to be more visible. If you are black, don't even consider having deep chemical peelings. They are sure to do more harm than good. You're also a bad candidate for this type of treatment if you have a family history or a personal tendency toward liver or kidney disease or keloidal scarring.

What Deep Chemical Peelings Can Do for You

If you are a fair-skinned blond with relatively dry skin, you can come away from this treatment with fantastic results. But the procedure is not a pleasant one. Ask the attending physician for a list of three or four patients who have undergone deep chemical peelings and talk to them about the experience. Be aware, however, that even those who have had deep chemical peels tend to minimize or forget what they went through because they are so pleased with the final results. In any case, prepare yourself for a pretty rough time.

There are cosmetic therapies such as collagen or silicone shots, or even face-lifts, that are designed to improve gross soft-tissue defects. Deep chemical peelings work well in tandem with these therapies to correct the fine defects which these other treatments cannot improve effectively by themselves, such as vertical lines above and below the lips, red spots, and other minor eyesores. Deep chemical peeling is also excellent by itself for the relatively young patient who has minimal facial sags but a few fine telltale lines, wrinkles, or skin discolorations that add years to an otherwise youthful appearance.

How Deep Chemical Peelings Work

The principal active agent for a deep chemical peel is phenol, a potent acid. The phenol is used to penetrate the epidermis and reach the dermis. There it eventually acts to add elastin to the skin's collagen by stimulating the activity of support-forming cells, which permanently raise the fine lines and wrinkles and make the face appear smoother and firmer.

To speed up and promote the phenol's penetration of the skin's outer layer, water, croton oil (an irritant), and a liquid soap are applied simultaneously with the active agent. The croton oil abets the absorption of phenol into the skin by destroying the epidermis, while the liquid soap adds surface tension to retard the coagulation of the phenol on the skin's topmost layer.

The immediate reaction is a whitening or bleaching effect on the face. This is because the phenol destroys the keratin, or coloring agent, in the skin layers as it penetrates. The epidermis, which is destroyed in the process, regenerates after seven days. The elastin-enhancing effect on the dermal collagen takes twice as long, or two weeks.

Keep in mind that this is a procedure that requires medical skill and experience from the physician for safety and best results. The right concentration and amount of phenol is vital to the treatment's success. There have been reports of sudden death during chemical peels resulting from kidney failure because of excessive absorption of phenol into the blood system. This can happen if too large a skin surface area is treated at one time. There is another potentially lethal side effect. The shock caused by the stinging sensation of phenol can produce an erratic heartbeat, which can precipitate ventricular cardiac arrest.

Because such potentially dangerous chemicals are involved, give all aspects of the treatment careful consideration before plunging ahead. This is not a casual undertaking, but a traumatic experience. It is also one that can be made worse by lack of preparation or foolhardy rashness.

If you decide to have a deep chemical peel, do not plan to do it just before or during the summer season. You need to avoid exposure to the sun for at least six weeks or more, which is almost impossible at that time of the year.

Undergoing a Deep Chemical Peel

A deep chemical peel is more frequently administered in a hospital but can be done in a dermatologist's office. Prior to actual treatment, a test application of phenol usually is swabbed onto a small area of the patient's skin to avert the possibility of a major negative reaction later. If no skin discoloration occurs, it is considered safe to proceed.

The face is cleaned thoroughly the evening before the treatment is scheduled and then washed again the next morning immediately prior to initiating the chemical peel. No general anesthesia is required. Instead a large dosage of Valium is given to the patient orally or by injection into the buttock. Next, the patient's face is swabbed with acetone to remove all the remaining skin oils. The application of acetone causes a stinging sensation followed by numbness. The face turns white. Wherever there are many fine wrinkles, the doctor dabs more acetone to obtain a smooth, white surface. At this point, the facial skin is ready for the phenol.

In applying the phenol, the doctor should spread out and stretch the wrinkled areas to make sure that the phenol covers and penetrates them. The deftness and skill with which this is done determines the treatment's ultimate success.

Another technique that ensures better results is overshooting the treatment area to prevent a noticeable demarcation line. This means that when doing the forehead, the doctor should dab some phenol over the hairline. If the lip area is being treated, some phenol should be applied over the lip borders onto the lips themselves, even though blistering is likely to occur.

The doctor applies the phenol to the face in stages—area by area—if more than one small part is being treated. After completing each facial segment, he or she tapes the area already treated with adhesive tape before going on to the next one. This acts to seal in the phenol and promote its penetration to the dermal collagen below, thereby maximizing the chances of long-lasting results. Treatment of the whole face takes approximately two and one-half to three hours, and requires some forty drops, or between two and three milliliters, of phenol.

The patient must rest in bed at least twenty-four to forty-eight hours, immediately following the procedure.

Here is what you can expect to experience after having a chemical peel.

You will start to feel considerable pain the day after the treatment is performed. The sensation is similar to that experienced when you receive a third-degree burn. The pain can be so excruciating that you may have to take some narcotics to withstand it.

The adhesive tape is removed on the second day following a chemical peel. Do not be shocked at what you will see. You face will look like raw liver: deep-red and bloody. At this point, application of thymol iodine powder begins. The substance, which resembles talcum powder, must be dusted onto any area that becomes moist for the next day or two.

On the fifth day after the treatment, you must apply some type of lubricating ointment—such as petroleum jelly or cold cream—to your face. The next day, the powdered skin layer, which is now a crust, comes off with the ointment. If your face is particularly hairy, wait one more day to allow the hair to loosen its grip before removing the crust. The crust will come off more easily then and you'll feel less pain.

Once the powdery crust is off, you can begin to wash your face with a mild soap, like Ivory, Basis, or Oilatum. You also can begin applying light makeup a week after the treatment, but wait another week or two at least before resuming application of regular makeup.

Do not expect the redness to fade quickly. It takes as long as six to eight weeks for the vivid coloration to slowly disappear and the skin to loosen up and become less taut. You may notice that any deeper lines and wrinkles you may have had are now less evident, an unexpected and pleasant bonus of the deep chemical peel.

As your face heals, you may see little whiteheads appear. These protrusions will go away by themselves.

The most common dissatisfaction experienced by chemical-peel patients is associated with the appearance of a demarcation line between untreated and treated areas. This can be avoided if the fair-skinned criterion is observed in treatment choice and if the hair and lip borders are overrun, as previously suggested.

Very rarely, there is some keloidal scarring from a deep chemical peel. Unfortunately, the occurrence cannot be predicted or prevented if the patient has not had a previous history or experience of this sort. In the few cases where the treatment has not proven effective at all, it can be repeated after two months have elapsed. However, most physicians recommend waiting at least a year and a half or two before trying again, and most doctors caution that if a deep chemical peel did not work for you the first time, it is unlikely that a subsequent try will be any more effective.

To maintain the unwrinkled look, you will probably need to undergo a deep chemical peeling treatment once every four or five years to keep the fine defects in check and retain your youthful appearance.

Mild Chemical Peels

If the idea of undergoing a deep chemical peel does not appeal to you, there is an alternative. It is a much less traumatic treatment that is highly effective for temporarily erasing fine lines and wrinkles. You will look younger and better for a period of three months to six months afterward.

The treatment, which takes only twenty minutes and costs about $100, can be done in a doctor's office. It involves a milder acid that is only 20 percent as potent as that used in a deep chemical peel. Painted onto your face, trichloroacetic acid turns your skin white. Your face becomes somewhat swollen for three or four days and then peels. During this time, be sure to keep out of the sun. In two or three weeks, you will look terrific. The slight swelling fills out tiny lines and plumps up little wrinkles to make your facial skin appear smoother and younger.

If you have a special occasion coming up and want to appear at your best, a mild chemical peel might be just the thing. Be sure to plan ahead. To obtain the maximum benefit, have it done at least three weeks prior to the big event.

An even milder version of the peeling treatment is offered. It is an acid peel equivalent to 3 percent the strength of a deep chemical peel.

This very mild chemical peel usually costs the same as a regular visit to the dermatologist. Administered in the doctor's office, it causes a slight burning sensation and some swelling. The effect rendered is that of a healthy suntan. Your face appears ruddy, smooth, and glowing.

Minor lines are filled out and little creases are pushed up by the temporary swelling. The beneficial effect is transient but noticeable. You will look healthier and younger for a few days, which can be well worth the moderate price.

8   SCRAPING AWAY

If you are overly sensitive about certain appearance-marring imperfections that make you feel old—fine vertical creases above your upper lip, or etched and crinkly flesh on the backs of your hands, or some unsightly blackheads or whiteheads around your eyes—and have tried unsuccessfully to have them cleared up or improved by other suggested therapies and remedies, there is a treatment of last resort that could work. Unfortunately, it is neither quick nor easy, nor is it cheap.

You will have to spend between $2000 and $4000 for something that will cause you considerable discomfort and inconvenience. You will look ghastly for about two or three months at least. But, ultimately, you could see a marked rejuvenation. Your skin could appear smoother, clearer, and sport a better color. You could look a lot better and more youthful, too.

This fairly drastic treatment is called *dermabra-*

sion. A tricky and painstakingly delicate procedure that involves the scraping away of the skin's entire top layer, or epidermis, it is the most radical of the cosmetic therapies for skin. Recent advances in medical equipment have made dermabrasions easier for the physician and safer for the patient. An innovative new hand-held instrument with diamond-coated edges allows lines and wrinkles to be sliced off mechanically by a doctor within minutes with minimal danger of irritating side effects or scarring.

Dermabrasions are not risk-free, however. Be advised that there are more malpractice suits associated with this procedure than with any other cosmetic corrective therapy. A contributing factor is on-the-job training of practicing cosmetic surgeons in the operating room. Because most physicians are not taught how to do dermabrasions in medical school, the majority of doctors who perform this type of surgery learn their craft and develop their skill by actually operating on patients.

The procedure, which requires only a local anesthetic, can be done in a doctor's office, although some experienced physicians prefer to have their patients hospitalized. The operation itself is fairly bloody and somewhat painful. A substantial amount of tolerance and patience is demanded of the patient, who must observe carefully a specified regimen of follow-up care during the protracted recovery period.

While the therapy eventually can make you look younger and more attractive by encouraging the growth of fresh new skin surface that is unblemished by age-caused or sun-induced imperfections, there is a chance you could end up looking no better, or even worse than before. In other words, despite all that you have to go through—the unpleasantness of the procedure and its aftermath—there is no guarantee of success.

Another drawback is that dermabrasions affect *only* the top skin layer. Since most wrinkles come from degeneration of underlying elastin and collagen supports, chances are your wrinkles eventually will reappear. So, further dermabrasions probably will be necessary to maintain the desired result. Most patients require repeated dermabrasion treatments every three to five years.

Considering what is involved, you should not undertake this therapy lightly. It is not for the squeamish or the unprepared. Know what you're getting yourself into and what you can expect in the way of improvement before you commit to having a dermabrasion. Weigh the potential benefits against the tally of financial, physical, and emotional costs. Base your decision on realistic expectations and a full understanding of all that a dermabrasion entails. Dermabrasions also are not appropriate for hemophiliacs or for people who suffer from herpes infections, warts, vitiligo, burn scars, or radiodermatitis, or for anyone who is prone to keloidal scarring.

What Dermabrasion Is and How It Works

A dermabrasion is a scraping down of the skin to do away with the surface imperfections—fine lines, wrinkles, and discolorations—that have developed from age and/or excessive exposure to the sun. It is the updated medical version of a beautifying treatment that has been practiced since time immemorial.

No doubt, cave men and women used to rub their faces with pumice stone to make themselves more appealing to the opposite sex. In the 1920s, cosmeticians began applying sandpaper to the face to literally buff up the appearance of the complexion. The 1950s saw the introduction of a specially designed rotary machine to allow quick, efficient removal of the skin layers. Then, in the 1970s, technological developments led to the diamond-coated, manually operated dermabraders that have significantly enhanced the precision, maneuverability, and control of the operating physician.

A dermabrasion takes the technique of epiabrading to its ultimate extreme, rejuvenating the skin by clearing off the damaged cells that cause a drab and uneven tone and texture. Further aging and deterioration of elderly or sun-damaged skin is halted by the resurfacing process. The taking away of the existing skin surface triggers the production of new skin cells in the underlying layers below, which eventually rise to populate the surface. Your complexion gets a fresh start with its new top coat of healthy cells. Skin feels better and appears younger-looking.

The daily shave is a very mild form of dermabrasion that provides beneficial conditioning for the face. Consider how baby-soft and smooth some old men's faces are. That is the effect of years and years of shaving with a razor blade. Along with unwanted hair, the razor blade slices off dead, damaged skin cells and other surface irregularities that mar the complexion and leaves the face smoother and clearer.

The trauma of the dermabrasion causes inflammation and edema, which, when they subside, produce appearance-enhancing effects. The swelling puffs out sags and crags, leaving the skin looking less wrinkled and lined. The heightened blood circulation adds a rosy blush, which gives the skin a healthy radiance and glow. After your face heals completely from the dermabrasion, your skin will feel softer and smoother. You will appear younger-looking and more attractive.

Getting a Dermabrasion

A dermabrasion is a very tricky and delicate procedure that demands great skill and experience. The surgeon must be deft and precise, knowing exactly how deep to cut for optimal results.

The aim of the surgery is to slice off everything above the borderline between the epidermis and the dermal layer below. If the doctor does not cut deep enough, the defects on the surface will appear unchanged; they will just be shallower. If the doctor cuts too deep and penetrates the dermis, permanent scarring and disfigurement can result.

Choosing the *right* doctor for this type of cosmetic surgery is especially crucial. Consult several physicians for their opinions before making your selection. Find out how frequently they perform dermabrasions and what type of equipment they use. Talk to some former dermabrasion patients, too, to get their reactions to the doctors and the surgery.

Diamond-coated manual dermabraders probably are your best bet for this type of surgery, since they permit more flexibility and control of the cutting edge. The machine comes with a range of abraders so that small skin areas can be treated individually with different grades of abrasiveness.

Another advantage of the manual dermabraders is that the abraders are disposable, which reduces significantly the chances of infection. Results, too, tend to be better. There are fewer reports of deleterious side effects or mishaps from dermabrasion surgery when manual dermabraders are used.

Still, there are risks with this type of cosmetic therapy, no matter how carefully it is performed. There is the chance your skin will wind up darker or lighter in spots. Black people tend to get white patches where skin is removed, so dermabrasion is not recommended for them. You also can contract a herpes infection because your skin is inflamed and more susceptible to the virus after the traumatic surgery. You might find yourself with milia, or little whiteheads, when your skin grows back. But these minor defects are only temporary and can be cleared away quickly with acne medicine. Even if you don't ordinarily have a tendency to get keloidal scars, there is the very slim chance that such thick scarring will occur.

If you are determined to have a dermabrasion despite the risks, do not have it done in the summer or in a sunny climate. Direct exposure to solar radiation must be scrupulously avoided for at least six months after the surgery. If you find you cannot avoid the sun, be sure to apply an effective sunscreen—a sunblock such as zinc oxide is even better—to protect the treated area.

Here is what to expect if you have a dermabrasion. After you arrive at the doctor's office or are checked into the hospital, you will be given some Benadryl or Valium to premedicate and relax you. When you feel somewhat drowsy, your skin will be cleansed and made ready for the operation.

The skin to be treated is frozen by spraying it with a topical anesthetic, Freon or Fluro-ethyl. This makes it white and hard, which allows the dermabrader to pass over the area and cut away smooth, even slices of skin. The areas are resprayed as often as needed to maintain the operative condition.

Because the entire top layer of skin is scraped

away, you will bleed a lot during the operation. After it is over, aluminum chloride will be applied to arrest the bleeding before you are bandaged.

You should rest in bed for at least twenty-four hours immediately following surgery. If hospitalized, you will be discharged the day after the operation.

Your skin will ooze under the bandages for the next five to ten days. Try to keep it as dry as possible. Some doctors recommend holding a hair dryer over the area as needed.

You will feel a crust form during the second week. At that point, the doctor will remove the bandages.

Be prepared for a shock. Your skin will look like raw liver. It will be very red and bloody. Do not expect a rapid transformation; your skin will heal very slowly. There will be a gradual improvement in your appearance over the next four to eight weeks.

When the recovery period is over, you should see a big difference in your skin. Its condition should be markedly improved, so that you look better and younger.

9   TAKING CARE

Aging is hard to accept. It is much easier to tolerate if you know you do not look as old as you really are. Fortunately, there are things you can do for yourself to temper both the severity and rapidity of aging, or at least conceal its deleterious effects, without resorting to the generally more expensive medical treatments discussed in the previous chapters.

By treating your skin properly, avoiding damaging sun rays, and applying appropriate protective creams, supplementary moisturizers, and beauty aids, you can keep your skin younger-looking longer. Once you know what to use, you will find most of the products you need to help you preserve a youthful appearance readily available without a prescription at drugstores, department stores, or supermarkets.

Cleansing

You have tiny organs under your skin called sebaceous glands that steadily secrete oil to maintain lubrication of the surface above and seal in existing moisture. As you age, however, the sebaceous glands slow down and produce less lubricant to smooth your skin and hold in moisture. That is why skin becomes drier and tougher as you get older.

Environment, too, can accelerate the drying-out process. Desert climates or water-robbing cooling or heating systems contribute significantly to skin dryness. Indoor environments that are partially to blame for drying out your skin can be adjusted. Install a humidifier in your office or home, buy some plants, or set out a shallow pan of water to add moisture content to air that is being drained of water by central heating or a drying ventilation system.

While there is relatively little that can be done to reduce the negative drying effects of aging and environment, there is a lot you can do to correct the dryness that is self-induced. When you cleanse your skin, soap dissolves the oils that have accumulated on the outer surface and washes them away. Meanwhile, down below, the sebaceous glands work hard to replenish the oil lost in the cleansing with fresh secretions. But if you scrub too often with soap, which is drying to skin, your sebaceous glands cannot possibly replace the amount of oil that is being stripped away in the cleansing process.

Long, hot baths or showers exacerbate skin dryness. Observe what happens after you soak your fingers in hot water for a long time. Their shriveled appearance is caused by dehydration. Hot water opens the pores, allowing moisture to evaporate rapidly out of the skin. The same effect occurs all over your body when you take a long hot shower or bath. The hotter the water, the wider your pores open and the quicker the moisture escapes. Hot water in combination with soap is very drying to skin.

So, if you find your skin is becoming excessively dry, before going out to invest in expensive moisturizers, try changing your bathing habits. Take shorter baths or showers in cooler water, use less soap, and see what happens.

Interestingly enough, the one thing that *can* moisturize your skin is water, and water alone. But only a brief dousing is required to irrigate thirsty skin. Taking a short lukewarm or cool bath or shower provides enough moisture for absorption by your skin without causing pores to open and allow the moisture to escape. By keeping your showers or baths brief and cool, your skin not only soaks up the moisture it needs, but—even more crucial—holds on to it.

Skin that is dry can benefit from the extra lubrication of a superfatted soap. These are soaps that contain extra fats and oils to help seal in the existing moisture in your skin. Keep in mind that even oil-laden soap still is drying to skin. That is because any soap, by its very nature, is drying. What the added oil does is to inhibit the drying effect, to a certain degree, by coating the skin with lubricant to prevent moisture from evaporating out of your skin.

Dry-skin soaps are available in all price ranges with an assortment of lubricating additives—glycerin, lanolin, petrolatum, and such oils as vegetable, mineral, or castor oil. Tone, by Armour Dial Inc., a floral-scented inexpensive soap that is sold in supermarkets and drugstores everywhere, is an effective cleanser for dry skin. It has an uncomplicated formula—pure soap plus coconut oil—and costs under a dollar. Also good are two moderately priced superfatted products you will find in pharmacies: Basis, by Beiersdorf Inc., with tallow and coconut oil; and scented or unscented Oilatum, by Stiefel Laboratories, with vegetable oil.

Transparent soaps have a softer consistency and more fat than their opaque counterparts. Because they consist mostly of glycerin, a colorless substance that dissolves easily in water, transparent bars melt faster and thus don't last as long as regular ones. Another drawback is that while high-fat glycerin soaps are gentle cleansers for dry skin, most of them contain tiny traces of nitrosamines, known carcinogens that can sometimes be absorbed through the skin.

As indicated earlier, there is a *right* way to cleanse your skin—that is, by aggressively rubbing the surface with an abrasive cloth or Buf-Puf (see pages 48–50). The technique is called *epidermabrasion*, and it improves the look and feel of the skin surface by sweeping off accumulated debris and damaged skin cells and stimulating blood circulation. The conditioning action evens out the texture and livens the tone, making skin smoother and more glowing. Dry, elderly skin can benefit from mild epidermabrasion using a moisturizing lotion instead of soap to lubricate the Buf-Puf or washcloth.

You also can achieve the beneficial effects of epidermabrasion by treating yourself to a facial mask. Dermatologically speaking, a facial mask is the mildest form of epidermabrasion. It gets rid of excess oils and other unsightly surface irregularities, heightens blood flow, and produces a slight skin irritation, which tightens your pores by swelling the cells that line them, tones your skin by gently peeling off the drab top layers, and puffs out unflattering lines and wrinkles.

By putting a glob of liquid on your face with your fingers or a brush, letting it set and peeling or rinsing off the hard cast-like mask, you clear your face of surface imperfections, smooth your skin, give your complexion a rosy glow, and make wrinkles and lines disappear, at least temporarily. The effect is not permanent, of course. The improvement achieved by a facial mask is short-lived and fades after a few days. Nevertheless, for an important occasion, a facial mask can be just the thing to give your appearance a real boost.

Facial masks are widely available in all price categories. Good choices in reasonably priced peel-off masks that perform well include Blue Mask, by Max Factor; Peel Away Mask, by Coty; and the quicker-drying Brush On, Peel Off Mask, by Helena Rubinstein. A more expensive but excellent peel-off mask is Fresh Skin, by Etherea. In reasonably priced rinse-off masks that are mild but effective, there are Medicated Masque by Bonne Bell and Masque Frappe by Dorothy Gray. Or, if you prefer the more costly clay-based rinse-off masks, take your choice among Etherea's Active Mud Masque, Princess Marcella Borghese's Clay Masque, or any of the beauty masks offered by Clinique, Chanel, Orlane, Lancôme, or Charles of the Ritz.

Moisturizing

Skin that is rough or cracked from age, excessive sun exposure, or other environmental conditions needs the extra lubrication provided by a moisturizer. To get the maximum benefit and protection out of a moisturizer, saturate your skin with water shortly before applying moisturizer to a still-damp surface. This means moisturizers should be dabbed onto your face as soon as you step out of the bath or shower and towel dry (women), or immediately after you shave (men). As far as the rest of your body is concerned, apply moisturizers where needed just after washing.

The timing is important because moisturizers are

formulated to lock in the water that is already inside your skin. As explained earlier in the discussion on cleansing, the key to skin moisturization is water. It is the water content of skin—not the inherent oil—that determines the degree of dryness.

You hydrate and add moisture to skin by showering, washing, or shaving. But retaining that water is critical to maintaining soft, smooth, and supple skin.

That is where oil figures in. The sebaceous glands secrete a sealing film of oil to coat the skin surface and prevent moisture from escaping out of the pores. Sometimes, however, the amount of oil you produce yourself is inadequate to do the job. This usually happens as you get older because your sebaceous glands gradually slow down and secrete less oil. As a result, skin becomes dry and rough. The parts of your body with fewer sebaceous glands—cheeks, hands, and legs—tend to dry out faster, particularly when they are exposed, which they are most of the time.

Dry skin gets flaky and feels coarse to the touch because it does not have enough self-produced oil to seal in moisture and prevent water loss. A moisturizer compensates for this deficiency by supplying a smoothing and protective emollient to stave off water loss. Some moisturizing products also include a water-attracting humectant to help keep skin soft by drawing in more moisture. The key ingredient in all moisturizers, then, is lubricating oil—natural or synthetic, common or exotic, animal or vegetable—to which humectants sometimes are added.

There are many excellent moisturizers to provide a sealing coat to help keep your skin from losing its moisture. Surprisingly, perhaps the best moisturizer of all is a product that isn't labeled as such. It is something that is cheap and readily available—unadulterated petroleum jelly, better known by the name Vaseline, the trademark of Chesebrough Pond's Inc.'s perennial best-seller. While the pale yellow stuff is not particularly appealing to use, it is a great skin protector. The invisible barrier it forms holds essential moisture within the skin, where it belongs. For best results, use Vaseline sparingly. Do not glob it on. Take a small amount and rub it well into your skin until it disappears.

If you find Vaseline esthetically distasteful or too greasy to handle, there are lots of other fine moisturizers on the market. A highly recommended, sensually pleasing formula that is inexpensive and sold everywhere is Nivea, by Beiersdorf Inc. It has what it takes—lanolin, petrolatum, and mineral oil—to effectively lock in skin moisture.

Another alternative is the reasonably priced Vaseline Intensive Care Lotion, by Chesebrough Pond's Inc. With lubricating glycerine, mineral oil, and cetyl alcohol, this smoothing lotion has a nongreasy consistency that is quickly absorbed by thirsty skin, leaving no sticky residue to make you feel uncomfortable.

If you like the idea of attracting more water into your dry skin, there are several reasonably priced moisturizers that feature water-absorbing synthetic urea. Among the choices are either one of Aquacare's highly effective formulas—Aquacare HP, with 10 percent urea, and Regular Aquacare, with 2 percent urea. Both have several lubricating ingredients—petrolatum, glycerin, lanolin, and mineral oil—to smooth your skin and lock in the added moisture. Other good bets are Dermassage Medicated Skin Lotion, by Westwood Pharmaceuticals, which contains lubricating lanolin and mineral oil in addition to urea; Carmol Ten (10 percent urea) and Carmol Twenty (20 percent urea); Nutraplus cream or ointment (10 percent urea); or Baby Soft Body Lotion, by Loves, Inc., with water-attracting urea and propylene glycol plus emollient oils to lock in your skin's moisture. There is also the highly effective Oil of Olay by Olay Company, Inc., a light silky smooth neutrally scented lotion that contains moisture-absorbent cholesterol to irrigate your thirsty skin and mineral oil to soften and protect it.

There also is a new class of so-called supermoisturizers, revolutionary products that work wonders to reverse the damage wrought on skin by age or excessive sun exposure. Besides the usual smoothing emollients, these concoctions contain special additives that promote the gradual regeneration of the skin surface to replace the original spotted, blemished, and bumpy one.

These are the A-hydroxy-acid moisturizers discussed above (see pages 51–53), which can rejuvenate skin by resurfacing it. They achieve their remarkable restorative effect by selectively destroying damaged cells that are responsible for the skin's bad tone and texture and simultaneously triggering the production of a new crop of healthy cells to replace them. Skin is treated to a new top coat, or stratum corneum, that gives it a fresh, healthier and younger look.

Because of their inherent therapeutic value, preparations with A-hydroxy acids definitely are the wave of the future in moisturizing products. Currently, there is only a limited choice of such products readily available in the marketplace. Many costly lines of skin-care products contain the highly beneficial alpha-hydroxy acids, but you can do better with previously mentioned Lacticare moisturizing lotion (see page 52), which is **much** cheaper.

Taking the Sun

Soaking up the sun is risky business. While glowing tans are temporarily attractive, getting them can take its toll on your skin if you are not careful. The effect of sun exposure is cumulative and irrevocable. Both premature aging and skin cancer are directly linked to the sun.

Elastin, the protein substance that supports your

skin and gives it a firm tone, can be destroyed gradually by overexposure to solar rays. When elastin gives way, flesh sinks and droops. Sags and wrinkles appear. Too much sun can upset the delicate molecular balance within your skin cells, causing unsightly lesions on your face or elsewhere on your body, or even skin cancer. Another deleterious effect from careless and excessive sun exposure is that skin can become blotched with unsightly brown patches and develop a rough, leathery texture.

This does not have to happen to you, however. A lot of people mistakenly think you have to get sunburned in order to tan; but a sunburn is not a preliminary step toward tanning. The popular misconception arises from the fact that you can burn and tan simultaneously. You see only the redness at first because it covers the tan until it heals. The tan becomes visible only after the effects of the sunburn disappear.

Tanning and burning are separate reactions of your skin to different ranges of solar radiation. Unlike tanning, which is a normal skin reaction, a sunburn is an abnormal skin reaction that leaves permanent damage. That is why you should protect your skin from the sunburn-causing radiation that can harm it. You can shield your skin from harmful solar rays and still get the tan you are after by using one of the many effective sunscreen products that are widely available.

Sunscreens allow tanning with a minimum of sunburn. They do this by absorbing most of the ultra-

violet light that causes sunburn while letting through
the rays that make you tan.

Two things are important in choosing a sunscreen: the Sun Protective Factor—that's the SPF
number on the package—and the active ingredient.
This critical information indicates how much protection the sunscreen gives (different skin types require
different amounts), and whether the product will
work effectively—some chemicals do the screening
job better than others.

The higher the SPF number on the sunscreen
product, the more protection it provides. This does
not mean you should automatically go for the item
with the highest SPF number, because all people do
not require the same strength of protection. Your skin
type and past experience in the sun determine the SPF
number you need.

If you have dark skin and usually tan easily without getting sunburned, you require minimal protection, or a sunscreen with an SPF 2. If you generally
tan and burn in about equal proportion, you need
moderate protection, or a sunscreen with an SPF 4 or
6. If you're relatively fair and usually burn easily and
tan with difficulty, you could use maximum protection, or a sunscreen with an SPF 8 or 10. And if you're
extremely fair and always burn without ever tanning,
you could benefit from the ultra protection of a sunscreen with an SPF 15.

The SPF number is a guide to the amount of time

you can safely soak up the sun's rays using a particular product, compared to no protection at all. It tells you how much of a defense—in terms of time multiples—the sunscreen provides against sunburn. Practically speaking, this means you can lie out in the sun two to fifteen times as long—depending on the SPF value of your sunscreen—absorbing the tanning rays without getting sunburned, as you could with unshielded skin.

The key ingredient to look for in a sunscreen is PABA—short for para amino benzoic acid—or any of its derivatives, like padimate. It is far and away the most effective screening agent. A couple of pointers about PABA: it performs best in low concentrations —no more than 5 percent; and it is most effective in an alcohol base. PABA loses some of its efficacy in oils, but performs well in lotions and gels, which generally are alcohol-based.

An excellent sunscreen for aging or dry skin is Eclipse 15 Sunscreen Lotion by Herbert Labs. It is reasonably priced and contains PABA for maximum protection against damaging ultraviolet rays and a built-in moisturizer—urea—to keep your skin from drying out. Other fine performers include PreSun 5% PABA Gel and PreSun 15 Sunscreen Lotion (Ultra), both by Westwood Pharmaceuticals; Sundown Sunscreens by Johnson & Johnson, with PABA and moisturizing emollients in all strengths with one exception—Sundown SPF 15 because it's a 7 percent PABA concentration; Sunguard Lotion by Dome

Laboratories with padimate and moisturizing emollients in an alcohol base; and Block Out Clear Lotion 10 Sunscreen by Sea & Ski, which has PABA in alcohol.

For people who don't spend their lives out in the sunshine, a sunscreen is imperative *only* for the first few days of sun exposure. You can cut down on your use of it once you develop a good tan. For people who either work outdoors or spend a good deal of time under the sun, sunscreen protection is necessary all the time.

For best results, be sure to apply your PABA-based sunscreen *before* you go out in the sun. Rub it well into your face, neck, hands, arms and anywhere else that is exposed. Make sure it is dry before venturing out under the rays.

Covering Up

If sun-caused or age-induced imperfections bother you and you are not interested in tampering with them to achieve permanent correction, you can do some cosmetic doctoring on your own. Skin discolorations, dark shadows, tiny lines, and little wrinkles can be covered up with the help of commercially prepared and widely sold concealers and antiwrinkle preparations.

Opaque and solid, concealers consist of mineral

oil or lanolin, talc, a heavy covering agent—like zinc oxide or titanium dioxide—and beeswax. Packaged in retractable dispensers, like lipsticks, they can be applied to cover up and lighten superficial imperfections on your face—unflattering dark shadows, little liver spots, and other sun-induced discolorations.

Just touch the stick to the area and blend the coloring into the surrounding skin. Top choices in concealing products include the inexpensive and well-formulated Erace by Max Factor; and two moderately priced alternatives—Highlight White Vanishing Stick by Revlon and Almay's Cover-Up Stick.

Antiwrinkle preparations, needless to say, cannot do away with wrinkles permanently or prevent them from appearing. What they can do is temporarily improve your appearance by making wrinkles look better or less noticeable. They achieve their short-lived effect through a combination of irritation and moisturization. The emollients and humectants they contain smooth and soften skin and the irritating agents produce a slight reaction that puffs out fine lines and wrinkles. Two good stick products in handy dispensers are Clinique's Wrinkle Stick and Etherea's Wrinkle Gel Stick. For those who prefer a cream, there's Dorothy Gray's Cellogen Moisturizing Hormone Cream or Helena Rubinstein's Pasteurized Face Cream Special.

Conclusion

By taking good care of your skin and protecting it from self-induced or environmentally caused dryness, discoloration, and roughness, you can stave off and delay unattractive aging. If you cleanse properly, supplement natural skin moisture as needed, and scrupulously provide the required protection against damaging sun rays, the premature appearance of wrinkles and lines can be averted.

Regular conditioning and the application of appropriate protective creams are the keys to preserving a youthful skin tone and texture. But remember, too, that even when unflattering aging signs do appear, it still is possible to get the medical help you need to treat yourself to younger skin.

INDEX